Praise for *Manage Your Menopau*

"It is fair to say that as a former primary care doctor, taught to believe that HRT [hormone replacement therapy] was the only solution for menopausal symptoms, I am now a total convert to 'managing your menopause naturally.' My own symptoms were not helped at all by several attempts with various forms of HRT, but after just three weeks of Maryon's program they had almost disappeared — and they have stayed away! Thank you, Maryon, and your team."

— **Dr. Vivienne McVey**, CEO, Virgin Care

"This is an excellent book providing an overall holistic approach to the management of menopause. It should prove to be very valuable to all women who are experiencing the myriad symptoms of menopause that they wish to manage in a nonmedicalized fashion, with practical and sensible tips that should be easy to implement. Even for those who wish to consider HRT, the advice Maryon Stewart provides is invaluable!"

— **Sushma Srikrishna**, MD, FRCOG, consultant urogynecologist,
King's College Hospital, London

"As doctors we haven't been educated about alternative routes through menopause. As many women want or need to manage naturally, it's important they have adequate knowledge. In *Manage Your Menopause Naturally*, Maryon Stewart brings together the world literature and, based on her successful approach that has been helping women overcome their symptoms for twenty-eight years, provides women with step-by-step instructions and tools to manage their perimenopause and menopause naturally, as well as future-proofing their health in the longer term."

— **Dr. Hina Pathak Sra**, MA (Hons), Oxon, MBBS, MRCOG,
Director, Harley Street Specialists

"Maryon Stewart is the go-to expert for resolving menopause challenges naturally, and I can't recommend her or this book highly enough. Her wisdom, expertise, heart, and compassion are unparalleled, and I'm so grateful this book will help her work reach more women. It's time to release the big fat lies about menopause and reclaim the second half of life with joy and enthusiasm. We deserve it, and Maryon is the perfect guide!"

— **Amy Ahlers**, author of *Big Fat Lies Women Tell Themselves*
and coauthor of *Reform Your Inner Mean Girl*

"As a menopause specialist, I know that hormone treatment is not always sufficient to treat menopausal symptoms. Women need holistic care, and many women are looking for a natural approach. Here, Maryon Stewart lays out her successful program, based on published medical research. In *Manage Your Menopause Naturally*, Maryon generously shares information from her Natural Menopause Solution so that women everywhere can use the knowledge to reclaim their well-being."

— Dr. Tania Adib, consultant gynecologist,
clinical lead of the Menopause Clinic, the Lister Hospital, London

"The important thing for me, as a practicing gynecologist, about Maryon's work is that it is evidence-based. This book is a fantastic place for every woman to start when faced with menopause and decisions about how to be their 'best self' for the next forty years. Maryon's balanced tone and obvious passion make her book a compelling read and her advice a pleasure to implement."

— Dr. Karen Morton, MA, MRCP, FRCOG, consultant gynecologist
and founder of Dr Morton's — The Medical Helpline©

MANAGE YOUR MENOPAUSE NATURALLY

MANAGE YOUR MENOPAUSE NATURALLY

The Six-Week Guide to Calming Hot Flashes
& Night Sweats, Getting Your Sex Drive Back,
Sharpening Memory & Reclaiming Well-Being

MARYON STEWART

Foreword by Emmanuela Wolloch, MD, FACOG

New World Library
Novato, California

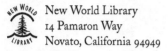

New World Library
14 Pamaron Way
Novato, California 94949

Text design by Tona Pearce Myers

Library of Congress Cataloging-in-Publication Data

Names: Stewart, Maryon, author.
Title: Manage your menopause naturally : the six-week guide to calming hot flashes and night sweats, getting your sex drive back, sharpening memory, and reclaiming well-being / Maryon Stewart ; foreword by Emmanuela Wolloch, MD, FACOG.
Description: Novato, California : New World Library, [2020] | Includes bibliographical references and index. | Summary: "A comprehensive six-week program for alleviating menopause-related health problems, without the use of pharmaceutical drugs. A series of questionnaires helps women assess which areas of their lives most need addressing. Issues discussed include concentration difficulties, mood swings, weight gain, skin complexion, and more."-- Provided by publisher.
Identifiers: LCCN 2020031717 (print) | LCCN 2020031718 (ebook) | ISBN 9781608686827 (paperback) | ISBN 9781608686834 (epub)
Subjects: LCSH: Menopause--Alternative treatment--Popular works. | Menopause--Nutritional aspects--Popular works.
Classification: LCC RG186 .S7469 2020 (print) | LCC RG186 (ebook) | DDC 618.1/75--dc23
LC record available at https://lccn.loc.gov/2020031717
LC ebook record available at https://lccn.loc.gov/2020031718

First printing, November 2020
ISBN 978-1-60868-682-7
Ebook ISBN 978-1-60868-683-4
Printed in Canada on 100% postconsumer-waste recycled paper

New World Library is proud to be a Gold Certified Environmentally Responsible Publisher. Publisher certification awarded by Green Press Initiative.

10   9   8   7   6   5   4   3   2

*To the wonderful women who were willing to share their very personal stories
in this book and on my website in the hope that they will help
millions of other women and their families around the world:*

Andrea Bauer
Fiona Bingham
Jo Brewis
Danielle Chamberlin
Lisa Finn
Anne Germany
Barbara Gustafson
Lorraine Hegarty
Joscelyn Bourne Leggett
Sharyn McLaughlin
Lilly Roads
Merle Shapiro
Joanne Simms
Gail Torr
Julie Whittaker
Helen Wilde

CONTENTS

FOREWORD

The menopause is a milestone in every woman's life. We may greet it with relief as an end to the tyranny of premenstrual syndrome, contraception, periods, and migraines, or we may regret the loss of fertility in the acknowledgment of aging. Most women feel a mixture of emotions, but what we really want is information about the process. We want to know what options are available so that we can make informed decisions about our future health and feel comfortable with our choices. This book is designed to help women do this.

Just as all women are emotionally, physically, and spiritually different, so are their experiences with menopause. Some women never experience a hot flash or night sweat, while others find their quality of life seriously compromised by hot flashes (or hot flushes, as we call them in the UK), night sweats, and a host of other debilitating symptoms that leave them feeling like shadows of their former selves, often scared and isolated.

Menopause is not a disease. It is a normal transition in the life of every woman who lives long enough to experience it. And regardless of the symptoms experienced before, during, or after menopause, it is a good time for a woman to take stock of her health and make changes that will help her to live a long, healthy, and happy life. After all, we can now expect to live as long after menopause as before menopause.

What women choose to do about their symptoms, or their health, at menopause is a highly individual decision. Whether or not a woman needs, or chooses, to use hormone therapy, all women should know what they can do to feel better — perhaps even better than before menopause.

With more than twenty-eight years of expertise in women's health, Maryon Stewart is bringing her highly successful menopause program from the United Kingdom to the United States. Women going through perimenopause and menopause now have a chance to improve their quality of life naturally through her Six-Week Natural Menopause Solution.

Manage Your Menopause Naturally helps women understand what to expect at menopause. More important, it enables women to make choices that will help them stay healthy and vital in the ensuing years. Health and vitality do not come in a bottle. They are reliant on the choices we make regarding our diet, exercise regimen, and other behaviors. Maryon Stewart's Natural Menopause Solution helps guide women to make healthy, science-based choices from perimenopause through to their postmenopausal years.

— Emmanuela Wolloch, MD, FACOG, holistic gynecologist

Introduction

WELCOME TO THE SECOND HALF OF YOUR LIFE

Making This the Time of Your Life

What if I told you that in a few weeks you could be feeling serene, sexy, wise, and calm, with harmonious hormones and free of your menopause symptoms? Wouldn't you want that? My Six-Week Natural Menopause Solution has already helped thousands of women improve their well-being. You can be next.

In 2020, more than 50 million women are going through menopause in the United States, and it's estimated that one billion women around the world will be experiencing menopause by 2025. That's 12 percent of the entire world population! You are certainly not alone. And while more than 75 percent of women will experience symptoms of menopause — such hot flashes, mood swings, difficulty concentrating, sleep problems, and loss of sex drive — for a decade or longer, 55 percent of those women won't do anything to try to alleviate them.

Often healthcare providers aren't stepping in to help, either. A Mayo Clinic study published in the *New England Journal of Medicine* in 2019 found that many doctors and gynecologists lack training or even a basic understanding of menopause management. Only 7 percent of them felt adequately educated to help women going through menopause. So women are simply left wondering what has hit them, understandably feeling that this is the beginning of the end.

It seems completely unfair to me that so many women of a certain age are experiencing misery unless they are armed with sufficient knowledge to do a U-turn. The information and tools to do that are out there. But conflicting advice and information overload on the internet often make it difficult to know where to start and whom to believe.

Many women who are savvy, straight-talking problem-solvers in other areas of life seem to roll over and become victims when it comes to problems with perimenopause and menopause. Why is it that so many of us accept discomfort and stress and assume it's all part of being a woman? It's a time when huge numbers of us lose ourselves and feel as if we've been taken over by an alien. It can be frightening and isolating: the symptoms are sometimes even too personal to discuss with our best friends.

While this book was in production, the COVID-19 pandemic hit, creating additional responsibilities, anxiety, stress, and fear that most of us had never anticipated. In addition to all the other challenges and difficulties women face at midlife, we have had to worry about our own health and that of our friends and families; about our income, jobs, and education; and about what the "new normal" will look like for those who survive the crisis. Many of us have been stressed by being confined in our homes and isolated from others, caring for family members twenty-four hours a day, and having to adapt to working and learning from home. Essential workers have faced extraordinary demands on their mental, physical, and emotional stamina. It's not surprising that many women feel they're being pushed into a danger zone, feeling unable to cope mentally.

We can't control external events, but we can take steps to improve our own well-being and resilience. Andrea Bauer, one of the women whose stories are featured in this book, hit the nail on the head when she told me, "Following your program I realized that I didn't need to degenerate at menopause, but instead, with adequate knowledge and support, I could regenerate." Even in a time of worldwide anxiety and uncertainty, that is so true.

Cutting through the Confusion and Taking Control

A few years ago, a friend of a friend posted on Facebook that she felt like she'd been hit by a steamroller. Her doctor had put her on hormone replacement therapy (HRT) to mitigate menopause symptoms, but the side effects were as bad as the symptoms.

After this woman's Facebook post, she was inundated with advice from friends offering "solutions." Hearing about them made me realize just how confused women are. Most of them warned her not to take hormones at any cost, because family members and friends had been diagnosed with cancer after taking them. Some of the suggestions involved gritting her teeth and bearing it without any treatment. Others recommended she try a range of supplements or creams, or make changes to her diet. None of them got it quite right. But one of her contacts suggested that she get in touch with me, because she knew that I had pioneered a scientifically based, nondrug approach that has been helping women overcome their symptoms for decades.

I am amazed, frustrated, and angry that women are still in the dark, fending for themselves, with so little direction at such a crucial time in their lives — especially when many of us have busy and challenging work and home lives. In my 2019 survey of 1,100 women, titled "What Women Want," 82 percent were hunting online for solutions to their suffering, without any clear road map or ability to distinguish good information from bad. In this survey, 37 percent of the women said they were given antidepressants for menopause; of these women, 80 percent felt this treatment was inappropriate. Although 41 percent were given hormone replacement therapy, 14 percent of those women didn't take it out of fear. Of those that did, 62 percent reported they came off it because of adverse side effects. Ninety percent of all the women in this survey said they would like information to manage their menopause naturally.

The health issues associated with menopause go beyond managing the symptoms that hit us at perimenopause and menopause. In the years that follow, as our estrogen levels decline, we are at greater risk of heart disease, dementia, and osteoporosis. One hundred years ago, when women didn't live long past the age of fifty, these were less significant concerns. But these days, when the big 5-0 is just the halfway mark for many of us, it's hugely important to keep ourselves in good shape and to avoid becoming reliant on a cocktail of drugs and hormones that often have adverse side effects. As a result, we can joyously embrace all the days we're blessed with, feeling confident that we're still in the driver's seat.

Most of the natural wellness books I have written over the years are fully medically referenced. (See the extensive reference section at the back of this book.) My drug-free approach is well supported by the medical literature. Much of that research might just as well be a secret, though. Women are often left in the dark during menopause, asking their doctors and friends for advice and not getting many answers other than suggestions of drug or hormone therapy, which at best should be considered a short-term solution. It's a scandal and very unfair for womankind, because there is an effective solution that can be tailored to your individual symptoms, lifestyle, and budget.

This Six-Week Natural Menopause Solution is based on the program my team and I pioneered at the Natural Health Advisory Service (NHAS), an organization I ran in the 1990s, which helped hundreds of thousands of women all over the world. There is no need to suffer alone or to be conned into taking products that don't even contain what they say on the label, or haven't been shown to be either safe or effective. With the right knowledge, women can easily overcome their symptoms and reclaim their well-being *naturally*.

Perhaps because women often put the needs of others before their own, many of us don't make time to look after ourselves properly. In addition to the physical symptoms we suffer from, the changes to our waistline and appearance occur so gradually that often it's not until one day when we glance in the mirror and get a shock that we realize just how far south we have traveled! Though you may be one of those women who dread aspects of this journey, I can assure you that women who have been through my Six-Week Natural Menopause Solution overwhelmingly regain their zest for life, get back into good shape, experience increased self-esteem and libido. Many end up feeling better than they can ever remember.

There's no need to suffer during menopause. There's an effective solution for you, and it will be my pleasure to help you feel better!

I feel passionately that women should be able to get proper direction at what can be a hugely scary stage in life. There is simply no reason to suffer when you can feel so good! I hope this book boosts your well-being now and in the future. You are most welcome to join one of the virtual classes I run at maryonstewart.com /masterclass, where I often answer questions live.

Navigating Perimenopause and Midlife Mayhem

When signs of perimenopause first appear, it's common to wake up in the morning feeling like life as you knew it is a dim and distant memory. Your hormones are in the driving seat, and you are left clinging on by your fingernails. Gone are the days when you rolled over in the mornings hoping your partner was in the mood for some fun. Instead of snuggling up for comfort and love, you are only too pleased to be on your own side of the bed, throwing off the covers as the heat overpowers you. When you cool down, you start to worry that having sex will be a nightmare, leaving you feeling sore instead of satisfied.

Repeated nights interrupted by drenching sweats leave you feeling overwhelmingly tired. Your skin takes on a pale hue and circles appear under your eyes, making you look like you haven't slept for weeks. You drag yourself out of bed to get on with your day, but you struggle because you have no energy. You have gained weight through comfort eating, and your clothes are too tight, while lack of exercise has made you despondent and depressed. Frequent, unannounced "power surges" make your face as red as a beet, and you feel like you are melting. You wonder where all this may be going. How will you cope? Should you seek advice? Take hormones? You go online to find some natural alternatives, but the overwhelming amount of information makes you feel even more confused than you already are. In the back of your mind you wonder whether your partner will be supportive or might get fed up with the significant change in your relationship. Some of the things that are happening to you may even be too embarrassing to discuss with close friends, so you sit in not-so-splendid isolation, wondering what comes next.

> By week 6 of Maryon's Natural Menopause Solution I was pretty much symptom-free. My vaginal tissues healed, and my libido returned, which delighted my husband. I feel really great again. I can't believe the difference. I'm so grateful.
>
> — Helen Wilde

These are the reasons I developed my Six-Week Natural Menopause Solution. It can take you from feeling stressed, washed out, irritable, tired, and confused and in hormonal turmoil to feeling sexy, wise, intuitive, turbocharged, and cool (what I call the midlife SWITCH), and brimming with happy hormones. That might seem a big stretch right now. Your first mission is to be trusting and come with me on a journey to reclaim your mojo and get back in the driving seat.

The Basics of Menopause

Menopause literally means the end of menstruation, although most of us use the word more loosely to describe the physical and mental changes that we experience in the years before and after this event. It generally happens any time between the ages of forty-five and fifty-five, with around fifty-one being the average.

At birth, our ovaries contain thousands of follicles, or egg sacs, in which egg cells ripen and develop. At puberty, our ovaries start to release an egg each month under the influence of two chemical messengers, or hormones, produced by the pituitary gland in the brain. These two hormones, follicle-stimulating hormone (FSH) and luteinizing hormone (LH), in turn trigger our ovaries to produce two more hormones, estrogen and progesterone, which are responsible for thickening the lining of the uterus in preparation for conception and pregnancy. If no egg is fertilized, estrogen and progesterone levels decline, and the egg, together with the built-up uterine lining, is shed. This accounts for the bleeding during a period.

As we move through our forties, the supply of eggs we were born with starts to run out, and our ovaries stop releasing an egg each month. This means we no longer produce so much progesterone and estrogen. Eventually, our ovaries run out of eggs altogether, progesterone production ceases, and estrogen levels fall to an all-time low. Because estrogen is required for many bodily functions besides reproduction — including maintaining strong bones, a sharp mind, and a healthy heart — it is inevitable that we feel the effects as our naturally occurring estrogen levels drop. Replacing the body's own estrogen with estrogens from plant sources not only replenishes our supply but also prevents the estrogen receptors in our cells from binding to estrogen-like chemicals in the environment (such as hormones used in meat production and some chemicals leached from plastics), which increase our risk of cancer.

Perimenopause

The body goes through a series of changes in the eight or so years leading up to menopause. These are known collectively as *perimenopause* (*peri* meaning "around"). The first sign that things are on the move is usually a change in the pattern of your periods. They may become irregular, longer or shorter, heavier or lighter. Other signs include hot flashes, night sweats, mood swings, loss of libido, loss of energy, sleepless nights, and difficulty concentrating, all of which may worsen over time.

Most of us are unprepared for perimenopause. For some women, it may simply be the inconvenience of never being sure when their period is going to arrive. If you are less fortunate, you may experience a worsening of PMS symptoms, as well as frequent mood swings and more "black" days.

PMS Meets Perimenopause

Premenstrual syndrome (PMS) refers to the physical and mental symptoms that occur just before the arrival of a period, then diminish or disappear shortly afterward, such as mood swings, bloating, food cravings, and digestive upset. Studies reveal that PMS is most prevalent in women in their thirties. But for some women, PMS never quite goes away. If your PMS bumps into the start of your menopause symptoms, which is quite common, then you have the worst of both worlds! In fact, due to the hormonal instability of perimenopause, PMS can become even worse.

Reliable research has found no consistent hormonal abnormality among PMS sufferers. Experts now think PMS may be caused by the undue sensitivity of the individual to the normal hormonal changes that take place in the second half of the menstrual cycle. This makes it much easier to see how PMS might fit in with some women's perimenopausal experience.

Some doctors may argue that the most successful treatments for PMS include those that effectively switch off the ovaries, blocking the menstrual cycle, but that's not what Mother Nature intended. Estrogen implants work amazingly well. But sadly, the benefit may not last, since the body adjusts to a new hormonal balance and the natural cycle re-imposes itself.

Our experience at the NHAS and evidence from other research show that PMS symptoms are often related to nutritional deficiencies, which can literally change the lenses through which we see the world. Billions of women around the world suffer nutritional deficiencies, even in wealthy regions. Symptoms can be reduced by improvements in diet, the use of certain nutritional supplements, and exercise. These changes can all influence female hormone function, the chemistry of the nervous system, general well-being, and physical fitness in a more gentle and effective way than hormonal treatment.

A study carried out by the NHAS looked at the relationship between previous PMS symptoms and current menopausal symptoms. We found some continuity between cognitive and emotional symptoms — such as anxiety, depression, confusion, and insomnia. However, there was little or no continuity of physical symptoms, such as hot flashes and night sweats. This lack of correlation suggests that menopause symptoms caused mainly by estrogen withdrawal are not greatly influenced by a history of PMS. Diet and lifestyle seem to make a big difference to many women's PMS symptoms, which is good news if you are going through mood changes at the time of menopause.

Early Menopause

About 1 percent of women experience menopause before the age of forty. This is known as premature menopause or premature ovarian failure (POF). You are more likely to have a premature menopause if

- Your ovaries are removed by surgery (oophorectomy), which sometimes happens with a hysterectomy if your ovaries are abnormal, or may be done to prevent the spread of endometriosis or ovarian or endometrial cancer.
- You have radiotherapy or chemotherapy for treatment of leukemia or cancer.
- You have a family history of early menopause or a chromosomal defect.
- You smoke. (Research shows that heavy smokers tend to reach menopause up to two years earlier than nonsmokers.)
- You had your last child before you were twenty-eight.
- You have never had children.
- You are short or underweight.
- Your diet is poor.

Have You Reached Menopause? Testing Your Hormone Levels

If your periods start to become erratic, or you haven't had a period for several months, you could be at the start of menopause. One way to find out is by measuring your level of follicle-stimulating hormone (FSH).

Before menopause, the normal range for FSH levels is up to eight units per liter (or mIU/mL, milliunits per milliliter). As you go into menopause, your levels of FSH may go as high as 100 units per liter. According to the North American Menopause Society, if a woman's FSH blood level is consistently 30 units per liter or higher and she has not had a period for a year, it's a sign that she has reached menopause. It usually remains at a high level for two years, or until your brain gets the message that your ovaries are no longer producing estrogen. At this point, FSH drops back to premenopausal levels.

Home kits for testing FSH levels in urine are available and can be ordered online. However, if you are still getting periods, your FSH levels will vary at different points in your cycle. For this reason, you will need to do the menopause home test twice, one week apart. If your FSH levels are high on only one of the tests, then it's likely that you haven't reached menopause. If both tests show a high reading, they confirm that you have arrived!

Midlife Switch

Fluctuating hormone levels may not be the only trigger of menopausal symptoms. Cumulative dietary and lifestyle factors can also play a significant part. Pregnancy and breastfeeding, as well as nutritional imbalances resulting from years of dieting, poor eating habits, or malabsorption, often leave us in a nutritionally depleted state as we reach midlife.

Menopause also tends to hit most of us at a psychological turning point, when natural fears about aging and the future start weighing on our minds. In addition, it's a time of life that often brings other challenges, such as the ups and downs of life with teenage children, caring for elderly relatives, relationship changes, trying to keep your career on track, or perhaps working outside the home for the first time in years. If, on top of all this, you have menopause to deal with, it's not surprising if you feel below par. The recent COVID-19 pandemic has placed even greater stresses and strains upon us.

Despite all the changes, it's important to keep things in perspective. Menopause needn't be the end of life as you once knew it; rather it marks the beginning of a new phase that can be just as exciting and rewarding as your earlier years. There's a lot you can do to make this transition smoother.

The Symptoms

Menopausal symptoms can be divided into three main groups:

1. Estrogen withdrawal symptoms
   - Hot flashes
   - Night sweats
   - Urinary incontinence
   - Recurring urinary tract infections
   - Loss of libido
   - Vaginal dryness
   - Painful sexual intercourse
2. Other physical symptoms
   - Aches and pains
   - Migraines and headaches
   - Fatigue
   - Constipation
   - Irritable bowel syndrome
3. Mental symptoms
   - Anxiety and panic attacks
   - Irritability

- Mood swings
- Depression
- Confusion
- Memory problems

What You Can Do

In recent years, by far the most popular treatment for menopausal symptoms has been hormone replacement therapy. However, studies connecting HRT with an increased risk of breast cancer and heart disease have seen this therapy fall from grace. Many women have tried to come off HRT and find an alternative for controlling their symptoms. Fortunately, you can overcome menopausal symptoms, as well as protect yourself against heart disease and osteoporosis in the longer term, without taking hormones.

Our latest audit of one hundred women on the 5-month NHAS Natural Menopause Program found that over 91 percent weaned themselves off HRT without any significant adverse effects. In addition, 66 percent of these women were completely or almost completely free of menopause symptoms within five and a half months of starting the program. A further 22 percent experienced some improvement in symptoms. The non-HRT users in particular experienced a dramatic reduction in the severity of their symptoms, with most going from severe to only mild symptoms. More than half the women also said their home life had improved and they were more productive at work.

I really never thought I would find the old me again, but I am so relieved and grateful that I have. I can think clearly now, work in my usual efficient way, and be there for my family with energy and enthusiasm rather than hiding my overwhelmed self away.

— Gail Torr

A wealth of published research shows that natural approaches, including using isoflavones (Mother Nature's estrogen), taking herbs like maca and St. John's wort, having acupuncture, and regular relaxation are effective and cost-effective ways of controlling menopause symptoms.

Getting Started

In this book I reveal the secrets to managing menopause naturally, allowing you to devise your own program to help you through the menopausal years. Key areas I focus on include:

- Replenishing estrogen levels by following a diet rich in naturally occurring plant phytoestrogens
- Boosting nutrient levels to help your brain chemistry and endocrine system to function normally
- Learning to relax, which can dramatically reduce hot flashes and help you feel more in control
- Losing weight without dieting
- Reducing stress
- Improving your fitness and mental health through regular exercise
- Building up bones and muscle
- Protecting your heart and lowering cholesterol levels
- Sharpening your brain
- Rekindling your libido
- Rebuilding your self-esteem
- Regaining your zest and vitality for life
- Experiencing the benefits of nutritional supplements, such as phytoestrogen-based, hormone-moderating supplements that have been scientifically tested.

Part I

MY SIX-WEEK
MENOPAUSE SOLUTION

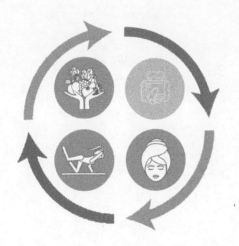

In an ideal world I would take you by the hand and guide you through my Six-Week Natural Menopause Solution week by week. The first week can be confusing, especially if you are experiencing brain fog and lacking sleep. So, before we start, I want to explain how the book is structured, tell you what to expect, and set out some rules that are important to your success with the program.

The six-week program came about after one million women watched my videos on Facebook in the space of twelve weeks. I realized I couldn't help them all individually, as I had helped my clients in my Harley Street clinic in London. My solution was to take the research-based tools I used in my five-month program, split them into six one-week online modules, and teach women how to manage their menopause naturally. I hadn't realized at the time that even this condensed version of the program would be enough to turn women's lives around.

The program involves the use of various tools, dietary changes, and nutritional supplements. I add information about all of these elements gradually, week by week, to avoid overload and to make it easy to understand the reasons behind the changes you're being asked to make. This means that starting out, I'm asking you to trust me and the recommendations I'm making; the reasons behind them will become clearer as we progress.

The first six chapters of the book correspond to the six weeks of the Natural Menopause Solution. In week 1 I identify many of the most common symptoms of menopause, explain their underlying causes, and offer a set of general dietary and lifestyle recommendations to follow. In week 2 we take a closer look at the role of diet in hormone function. Since nutritional deficiencies contribute to a wide range of symptoms we experience at midlife, we look at ways to detect and correct them. In week 3 we look at the naturally occurring forms of estrogen that Mother Nature provides from plants and learn how we can use these to fool our brain into thinking that we once again have good amounts of circulating estrogen, alleviating symptoms like hot flashes and night sweats. In week 4 we focus on the many safe and well-researched natural remedies that exist for common menopause symptoms, so that you can choose the supplements that best meet your needs. We also explore options to make sure we're getting regular exercise and finding ways to relax. In week 5 we home in on coping with stress, improving sleep, and putting sex back on the menu. In week 6, and in the chapters in part 2 of the book, we look at wisdom, staying positive, complementary therapies, and ways to nurture and protect our health for decades to come.

Part 3 of the book contains various tools and resources to support you in following the program. These include meal plans, a selection of healthy recipes for those who like cooking, and recommendations for healthy store-bought options for those who don't. A list of foods containing significant amounts of important nutrients will help you select foods you enjoy while making your diet more nutrient dense.

Part 3 also includes tools for recording how you're feeling and tracking your progress. When you start the program, fill out the Natural Menopause Solution worksheet; you'll find it a valuable reference as you check in with yourself during the program. Throughout the six weeks, fill out the diet and symptom diaries. It's important to keep these up to date. They are a great source of information and motivation

As you go through each chapter of the book, make a note of the action points you need to follow. By the time you have finished the six weeks, you will have your own personally tailored program.

Nine Rules for Success (and Four Tips)

The Six-Week Natural Menopause Solution offers a lot of flexibility in tailoring recommendations to your personal needs, but there are a few rules you need to stick to in order to benefit from it:

1. Follow the program from week to week in real time, with one exception: review the nutritional supplement information in chapter 4 during the first week and choose the supplements that you feel will benefit you.
2. Stick to the dietary recommendations as if your life depends on it. Following the recommendations on some days and not others won't produce the gains you are hoping for. Don't skip meals.
3. Record all the recommendations you are going to be following in the My Natural Menopause Solution worksheet on page 232 and review them each week to make sure you're on track.
4. Take the recommended supplements for your symptoms without substitutions, unless medically indicated.

5. Make time for daily relaxation, as it will help control hot flashes, ease anxiety and brain fog, calm your bowels, and help your body cope with stress.

6. If you don't already exercise regularly, gradually develop an exercise routine following the instructions in chapter 4.

7. Only shop for food when you have a full tummy, to avoid making impulse purchases of less healthy items.

8. Only keep food that's on the menu in the house or in your office.

9. List everything you eat and drink in the Diet Diary (page 235) to keep yourself accountable.

Tips for Sticking with the Program

1. Expect withdrawal symptoms in the first week; you may feel worse before you feel better.

2. Plan your menus before you go shopping.

3. Stock up with phytoestrogen-rich foods, including snacks.

4. Ensure that you consume small amounts of isoflavones often throughout the day and evening.

I don't have a magic wand — just a really effective program that works when women follow it to the letter. It takes time to see the gains. The first few days may be challenging as you make changes to your diet and lifestyle: some women experience caffeine withdrawal symptoms, for example, which can include headaches and mild anxiety, but they pass in a few days. If you work during the week, you might want to start the program on a weekend so that you can rest and hide away if you are not feeling your best.

While all the techniques and supplements I recommend are safe and natural, if you are receiving medical treatment, or if you're experiencing debilitating symptoms that might be caused by an underlying medical condition, it's important to consult your doctor to get approval of these recommendations and ensure that they are compatible with any medication you may be taking.

Chapter 1

WEEK ONE

Jump-Starting Your Menopause Solution

We each have our own journey through menopause. Some women sail through and honestly wonder what all the fuss was about. But for many others, the hormonal ups and downs result in bodily changes and unwanted symptoms that disrupt their lives and result in utter misery.

Constant hot flashes during the day and sweats at night can leave you exhausted, disoriented, and despondent. Vaginal dryness and reduced libido can wreck your sex life, while headaches, chronic insomnia, and woolly-headedness can make you wonder if life will ever be the same again.

The good news is that these are menopausal moments — and like all moments, they will pass. My goal is to help you fast-track the process naturally with simple diet and lifestyle adjustments. The only side effect will be that you feel more like yourself, or possibly a whole lot better!

Though some of the symptoms of menopause can take weeks or even months to ease, in week 1 of the Six-Week Natural Menopause Solution we start by alleviating the symptoms you can do something about right away, from reducing hot flashes and night sweats to easing achy joints and painful sex. (Check out the cheat sheet listing symptoms, possible causes, and recommended solutions on page 35.) I want you to start feeling better immediately, and I know from experience that once women get a taste of how good their bodies and minds can feel, it motivates them to keep going.

Quiz: Assess Your Symptoms

This quiz will help you identify your main problems. Based on your responses, I will show you how to tailor your plan based on your own individual needs. Check all of the symptoms below that you're currently experiencing. Give honest, spontaneous answers.

- ❑ Hot flashes
- ❑ Night sweats
- ❑ Vaginal dryness
- ❑ Anxiety
- ❑ Irregular or heavy periods
- ❑ Frequent need to urinate
- ❑ Stress incontinence (bladder leakage when laughing, coughing, or sneezing)
- ❑ Forgetfulness
- ❑ Depression
- ❑ Loss of confidence
- ❑ Trouble concentrating
- ❑ Difficulty sleeping
- ❑ Aches and joint pain
- ❑ Heart palpitations
- ❑ Panic attacks
- ❑ Headaches
- ❑ Loss of sex drive
- ❑ Painful sex
- ❑ Mood swings
- ❑ Fatigue
- ❑ Weight gain
- ❑ Bloating

If you checked more than three items, then my Six-Week Natural Menopause Solution can help you manage your particular perimenopause or menopause symptoms and, if necessary, provide you with a tried-and-tested way to wean yourself off hormone replacement therapy (HRT) without any side effects. You will restore your self-esteem, rekindle your libido, resurrect your memory, recharge your batteries, and regain your zest for life, all in the space of a few short weeks, by following a program that has helped literally hundreds of thousands of women worldwide over the past twenty-seven years.

Going Natural

My approach offers a simple, workable, and enjoyable way of alleviating symptoms during perimenopause and beyond. It is based on sound, published scientific research (see the medical references at the back of the book). Its effectiveness astounds most clients.

During my years at the Natural Health Advisory Service (NHAS), we conducted several research projects measuring levels of nutrients in women at different stages of their lives. The results suggested that falling levels of estrogen are not the only trigger of menopausal symptoms. Diet and lifestyle also play an important part. Levels of some nutrients drop naturally as we age. By the time many women reach menopause, they are running on two cylinders instead of four. Women who are not in a good nutritional or physiological state are likely to suffer more severe menopause symptoms and face poorer long-term health prospects.

My Six-Week Natural Menopause Solution includes five approaches to overcoming perimenopause and menopause symptoms:

- Getting nutrient levels back into an optimum range
- Using natural plant-based estrogen compounds that bind to the estrogen receptors in our cells to fool the brain into believing we once again have normal circulating levels of estrogen
- Taking standardized nutritional supplements that have been proven both safe and effective
- Exercising regularly to keep our metabolism ticking over and release endorphins, our feel-good hormones
- Doing a session of relaxation daily to keep cool, calm, and relaxed

My six-week plan includes explanations of why common symptoms occur, nutritional deficiencies that can contribute to symptoms, and action plans to address specific symptoms. Chapter 4 includes a list of supplements that have been medically proven to soothe menopause symptoms and help boost your overall health and well-being. Combine these recommendations with the meal plans and delicious recipes in part 3 to make sure you meet your body's nutritional needs. Also included is information on the nutritional content of many foods.

As soon as you start addressing your body's needs, symptoms like hot flashes, night sweats, depression, headaches, aches and pains, insomnia, mood swings, and anxiety will begin to subside. You will also start lowering your risk for many life-disrupting (and often life-threatening) conditions, including heart disease, osteoporosis, estrogen-related cancers (such as breast cancer), kidney problems, memory loss, and dementia.

Barbara's Story

Barbara is a fifty-three-year-old multimedia expert and award-winning filmmaker from Austin, Texas. When she first approached me for help, she was unable to sleep and suffering with anxiety and brain fog.

I was so afraid that I was getting dementia, because my short-term memory was shot. I hated the aging process — and myself, at times. I dreaded getting up in the morning, and at night my brain would go a hundred miles a minute, so I never felt rested.

I suffered with menopause symptoms for five years. I felt desperately anxious, especially because of the brain fog. It made me feel scared and totally incompetent. Despite the fact that I was always yo-yo dieting, I was grossed out about my weight gain so I distanced myself from my husband. I felt moody, I couldn't sleep either, and all of this gave me very low self-esteem, and I certainly didn't feel like having any physical contact.

Loss of concentration was another disconcerting symptom. This left me feeling even more anxious, as I couldn't maintain my train of thought while I was working, and that's crucial to the success of my work. My doctor thought I had ADD (attention deficit disorder) and prescribed a high dose of Adderall, which was unsustainable as it gave me extreme headaches.

I hadn't realized I was going through perimenopause.

Within the first few weeks of being on the Six-Week Menopause Solution I began losing weight. My brain fog disappeared a bit later, and sleep got gradually better. The difference for me is like the difference between night and day. I am now probably my most creative in years and can write with ease and actually enjoy my work. Falling asleep is not a problem, which is great considering my work schedule. I can also think clearly without scary brain fog. I feel like I am in charge and have a more positive body image.

I look forward to the future and actually like myself again. I have only begun this next chapter in my life, and from what I can see it's going to be a doozy. My dreams and aspirations are taking shape. Now, instead of being scared, I can't wait for the next adventure.

A New You

Having worked with hundreds of thousands of women over the years, I have witnessed wonderful transformations as women regain their quality of health, confidence, and self-esteem. The women who share their experiences for this book are just a few typical examples.

Their stories show you that you are not suffering alone and that the end of your symptoms is in sight. This is your chance for a happy and healthy new beginning!

Joscelyn's Story

Joscelyn was a dynamic professional woman who was struggling to cope with the disruptions to her life caused by her menopause symptoms.

When I reached approximately forty-five, I started to notice that I was increasingly experiencing dark moods (I am naturally a cheerful person) and would often have (as I now call them) "black" days. At the time, I had a busy career running a print and design company with my husband, and my responsibility was to pull work in. Naturally this meant a lot of contact with customers, both on the phone and face to face. On black days, I could not cope with talking to anyone and would often find myself at home on the sofa, comfort eating, watching TV, or sleeping.

Eventually, after about two years of trying to cope, I found Maryon Stewart on a Health TV channel. By this time I was desperate for help. I was putting on weight and becoming obsessed with food, experiencing increased mood swings, and feeling very run down and constantly tired.

I decided to get in touch with Maryon. At first I thought following the recommendations would be really tough (especially the alcohol side of things!), but I was so desperate to pick myself up, I knew I had to stick with it. My system was very low, and it took a few weeks before I started to see results, but following Maryon's advice and increasing my intake of isoflavones and phytoestrogens, I soon found that I was not craving food as I had previously. I have since introduced many of the foods that I'd eliminated back into my diet. However, I have learned to manage my diet in accordance with my menopause and ensure I focus on the isoflavones and phytoestrogens to stay on track.

It has literally been one of the best things I have ever done, and I will always be grateful for the sound advice and support.

A Quick-Start Guide to Managing Common Symptoms

Let's look at what causes menopause symptoms and how you can help yourself in the short term. Because some symptoms are interrelated, you may find that as you treat one, the others also improve. This is not an exhaustive list of symptoms; see the cheat sheet on page 35 for information on other common symptoms and advice on how to manage them.

Hot Flashes

Hot flashes and night sweats can be debilitating. More than 80 percent of women are affected by hot flashes at some point. They may start long before you stop menstruating and continue for several years afterward. Experts don't know for sure what causes them, but it's thought that a lack of estrogen may affect the hypothalamus — the region of the brain that controls body temperature.

The frequency, duration, and intensity of hot flashes vary from one person to another. You may get several a day or be plagued constantly, day and night. They may last from a few seconds to several minutes. (The average is four minutes.) As well as the sudden rush of heat, you may experience a racing heart, dizziness, anxiety, and irritability.

Night sweats are severe versions of hot flashes that can cause you to wake up drenched in perspiration. You may even have to change your pajamas and sheets.

If you're woken up this way, night after night, you're bound to feel exhausted. Worse, because physical contact with a partner can trigger a hot flash, many women avoid it, which can lead to feelings of rejection and relationship problems. Here are some ways to feel better fast.

Cooling Your Hot Flashes

- Don't be embarrassed by a hot flash.
- The moment you feel one coming on, stop what you're doing. Take several slow, deep breaths and try to relax. This may help reduce the severity of the hot flash.
- If possible, drink a glass of cold water and sit calmly until it passes.
- Wear layers that you can easily take off when you feel yourself getting hot. Clothes made of natural fibers, such as cotton, help your skin breathe.
- Keep your bedroom cool at night and put a fan, wet wipes, and a cold drink by your bed.

- Use cotton bedlinens and pajamas.
- Eat small, frequent meals. The heat generated by digesting a large meal can sometimes bring on a hot flash.
- Exercise regularly. Being in good shape reduces your propensity to sweat and reduces hot flashes.
- Don't smoke. Research shows it increases the risk of overheating.
- Include plenty of phytoestrogens in your diet. (See the list of phytoestrogen-rich foods on page 60.)
- Try scientifically based supplements, like Promensil and Femmenessence MacaPause, which have been shown to reduce or even eliminate hot flashes and night sweats.

Did You Know?

It's likely the hot surges you experience are the result of your brain trying to kick-start your ovaries into producing estrogen. Ovarian function does not decline in a straight line, which means that estrogen levels — and the severity of hot flashes — can fluctuate.

Headaches

Headaches and migraines are common during menopause and may be caused in part by changing body temperature, tiredness due to hot flashes, sleeplessness, or general stress and anxiety. Migraines can also be affected by falling estrogen levels and may either diminish or worsen during menopause.

Managing Headaches

- Practice relaxation techniques, like deep breathing.
- Exercise regularly. It helps increase blood flow to the brain, which may alleviate headaches.
- Headaches are sometimes caused by low blood sugar. Eating a wholesome snack before bed can help keep your blood sugar level balanced and prevent you from waking up with a headache.
- Try complementary therapies, such as massage and acupuncture.

- Practice tapping exercises (see page 147), an acupressure technique that can eliminate pain.

Painful Sex

Lack of estrogen causes a decrease in the mucus-producing cells in the lining of the vagina, making it thin and dry. As a result, sex can become uncomfortable, and in some cases painful. A decrease in muscle tone and a resulting reduction in the blood supply to the urogenital area may also be a factor. The good news is that this is reversible through diet, supplements, and other approaches.

Jump-Starting Your Sex Life

- Try Membrasin® SBA24® capsules (known as Omega 7 SBA24 in the UK) to help alleviate vaginal dryness and discomfort (see page 82).
- Try products like Membrasin® Vaginal Vitality Cream and other personal lubricants, which can make sex much more comfortable and pleasurable.
- Have regular sex. As counterintuitive as it sounds, it can help with vaginal lubrication. And spend plenty of time on foreplay!
- Do pelvic floor exercises (also known as Kegel exercises) to strengthen the muscles and increase blood flow. In addition to doing the simple exercise described below, look for Michele Kenway's instructive videos on YouTube, which range from basic to more advanced pelvic floor exercises.

WORKING YOUR PELVIC FLOOR MUSCLES

1. Sit with your eyes closed and think about the muscles you'd use to stop urine flow.
2. Contract those muscles as tightly as possible.
3. Hold for several seconds. It should feel like the muscles are lifting in and up.
4. Relax for several seconds, then repeat once. Do the exercise 10 to 15 times a day.

Mood Swings

Depression, irritability, and anxiety are common menopausal symptoms that are probably caused by the hormonal and physical changes you are going through (just as teenagers get moody when they experience the hormonal roller coaster of puberty). You may find yourself weeping for no obvious reason, being unable to make up your mind about the smallest things, or feeling panicky at the thought of tackling something you'd normally take in stride. It is important to realize that these feelings are normal and will pass, although it may take time. If you are experiencing deep depression and even suicidal thoughts, though, it's important to check in with your medical team.

Evening Out Mood Swings

- Don't keep your feelings bottled up — talk about them with a friend, a family member, or your partner.
- Follow a phytoestrogen-rich diet. (You'll find a list of convenience foods that contain good doses of them on page 217.)
- Exercise regularly. There's good evidence that being active elevates mood.
- Try doing a yoga session each day, maybe using online videos for guidance if you haven't done yoga before. Yoga with Adriene, on YouTube, offers a free thirty-day course that is a great place to begin.
- Practice relaxation techniques like meditation, or try a using a guided meditation app.
- Keep a list of things you're grateful for. Looking over it can lift your spirits and help you keep things in perspective.
- Watch a fun movie.
- Dance to your favorite music.
- Practice mindfulness and mindful breathing to keep yourself grounded and in the moment (see page 91).

Insomnia

A succession of sleepless nights can be severely debilitating, so it's important to address insomnia as soon as you can. Common causes include night sweats, anxiety, and having to get up in the night to go to the bathroom. Poor or disturbed sleep can trigger many other symptoms, such as depression and irritability, so sleeping better may also help improve your mood.

Getting a Better Night's Sleep

- Try relaxation techniques, especially right before bed (see page 90).
- Exercise regularly. It's been shown to improve the quality of sleep.
- Have a cup of chamomile or valerian tea or warm soy milk before bed.
- Avoid caffeinated drinks completely, as the caffeine can act as a stimulant and keep you awake. These include, tea, coffee, cola drinks, and hot chocolate.
- Listen to soothing music. It can help you relax and sleep more soundly.
- Try not to take worries to bed with you. Jot down anything that's bothering you to get it off your mind, and then consciously distance yourself from any troubles by focusing on something you find soothing.
- Avoid watching, reading, or listening to anything too stimulating in the evening, and avoid electronic screens (laptops, tablets, and smartphones) at least an hour before bed. Research shows that the blue light they emit can disrupt sleep.
- If you frequently wake during the night, taking the herb valerian can help you get back to sleep. If you find it hard to get to sleep, try taking valerian half an hour before you go to bed.
- Try the Pzizz Sleep app (see chapter 4).

Dry Skin

Many women start to notice their skin becoming drier around the time of menopause. You may also see an increase in wrinkles. Both are due to the effect of lowered estrogen levels on collagen, the structural protein in skin that keeps it firm and elastic. Keeping your skin well hydrated and eating plenty of foods rich in phytoestrogens can counteract dryness and fine lines.

Treating Dry Skin

- Moisturize, moisturize, moisturize! Look for plant-based products with no artificial chemicals. There are many lovely brands to choose from.
- Protect your skin from the sun's damaging UV rays by applying sunscreen with an SPF of at least 15 — particularly on your face, neck, and hands.

- Drink at least eight glasses of water daily to hydrate skin from the inside out.
- Regularly exfoliate your skin to remove dead skin cells and help your moisturizer penetrate skin more readily.
- Eat plenty of oily fish rich in omega-3 essential fatty acids (EFAs), such as salmon and sardines. These healthy fats help keep skin soft and smooth.
- Consider taking an omega-3 supplement.
- Try taking the natural supplement Equelle, containing S-Equol. In a study of 101 postmenopausal women, this soy-based product was shown to significantly reduce the depth of wrinkles after twelve weeks.

Panic Attacks and Palpitations

Women often experience panic attacks and even heart palpitations during menopause, even if they've never really been bothered by them before. These symptoms may come on suddenly, sometimes just prior to a hot flash, and be very frightening. One of the participants in my program reported that she had been taken to hospital five times in four weeks by ambulance while on holiday in Australia, as she thought she was having a heart attack. Doctors found no irregularities, and it turned out that her symptoms were related to menopause. After a few weeks on the Six-Week Natural Menopause Solution, once her "midlife refuel" was under way, her symptoms disappeared and never returned.

If you do experience cardiac symptoms, it's best to get them checked out by your doctor, for peace of mind if nothing else.

What is it about menopause that can cause or aggravate these symptoms? When hormone levels fluctuate, the brain sends a message to the hormone-producing adrenal glands, which can cause an adrenaline surge, part of the body's flight-or-fight response. A survey by the NHAS of one thousand clients found that 91 percent of women had suffered anxiety before their periods, and in severe cases had panic attacks and palpitations leading up to their periods. These symptoms can get worse as we age, because falling nutrient levels can impede normal hormone function. Once your nutrient levels and hormones are back in balance, your sense of well-being will likely return.

Easing Palpitations and Panicky Feelings

- Eliminate caffeine from your diet. Even teas, coffee, or soft drinks labeled as decaffeinated may contain enough residual caffeine to cause anxiety.

- Eat regular, wholesome meals and snacks to provide your brain and nervous system with a constant supply of nutrients.
- Minimize your consumption of alcohol, as it impedes the absorption of many important nutrients and can leave you feeling anxious.
- Don't smoke. Nicotine may seem to have a calming effect, but it is also a stimulant that should be avoided.
- When you begin feeling anxious, take a few slow, deep breaths and mindfully bring your attention to the moment. Repeating calming affirmations can be helpful at this point, as can focusing on something beautiful, like a flower or one of your favorite pictures.
- Practice formal relaxation or meditation each day.
- Use the Pzizz app to help you calm down when you feel anxiety building (see chapter 4).
- Take a good broad-spectrum multivitamin and mineral supplement each day, like Gynovite Plus or Fema 45+ (in the UK), which has been shown to boost nutrient levels and calm anxiety.
- Try taking valerian supplements to help you feel calmer, and rhodiola to reduce levels of the stress hormone cortisol. These adaptogenic herbs help your body deal with an elevated stress response (see page 82).

Fiona's Story

When Fiona first approached me for help she was forty-seven. She was scared by her extreme brain fog, especially as she had consulted several doctors who suggested she might have dementia.

I started to lose myself at the age of thirty-seven. For ten years I felt progressively worse before I realized it was due to menopause. My memory went blank, and I couldn't sleep. I had terrible aches and pains and body stiffness. I suffered palpitations, sometimes up to five episodes in an hour, and the heat permeating from my body made me feel unattractive and claustrophobic. My periods suddenly became a major disruption to my life, and I felt anxious and irritable most of the time. My confidence was very low, and I felt confused and afraid when my mind failed me, as it did on many occasions. Plus, I had severe constipation and bloating. My doctor, who rolled his eyes when I suggested it might be menopause, put me on Microgynon [oral contraceptives] to manage my periods, gave me some sleeping tablets, and referred me for a sleep apnea test and an ECG before diagnosing stress and advising I adjust my work-life balance.

Towards the end of it all I felt so ill, it was as if my brain had died. The brain fog was so severe, there was no point writing myself a note, because I wouldn't remember where I'd put it. Inevitably, I cut down on work and eventually left the workplace because I couldn't cope. If I had stayed, I know I would have cracked and had an incredibly public meltdown, as I was so overwhelmed. I can understand why women feel there is no point to living at this stage in their lives.

It was a sleep apnea nurse who was the first person to agree that my symptoms might be related to menopause, so I plucked up the courage and insisted my doctor measure my follicle-stimulating hormone, which had never been measured during my ten-year-long nightmare. I wasn't too surprised to find out it was elevated beyond belief. It confirmed I was in the middle of menopause. I was put on HRT, which I thought would be the answer, but I had unbearable side effects. Although it controlled the heat and palpitations, I put on masses of weight, still felt bloated, had chronic indigestion, vaginal bleeding, and headaches. Even though I began to sleep through the night, I was overcome with exhaustion. HRT also did nothing for the brain fog. On the advice of my doctor, after five months of nonstop bleeding, I stopped taking HRT. The effect was catastrophic: every symptom returned, and I hit rock bottom.

I found Maryon Stewart on Facebook and was interested in her years of experience helping women overcome menopause naturally. I enrolled in her Six-Week Natural Menopause Solution in June and made the changes she suggested to my diet and lifestyle, and I took some supplements that have been shown in clinical trials to help. I now feel like a different person. I feel like me again. I sleep. I wake up feeling refreshed. I'm clear-headed and no longer have brain fog. I no longer have bloating or constipation. I am able to work, and I'm even managing a house move now, which I couldn't have even thought about before.

I find it outrageous that my symptoms were so easily controlled by natural measures that are based on published research and don't have any side effects, yet most doctors are not familiar with them. It's beyond sad that women are left to suffer in this way. So many relationships are wrecked by menopause symptoms, and it's such a waste of talent in the workplace.

Aching Joints

Falling estrogen levels result in reduced lubrication in our joints. In addition, a lack of essential nutrients can cause degeneration and result in creaking bones and aching joints, especially first thing in the morning. Here are some tips for reducing pain and increasing mobility.

Soothing Aching Joints

- Eat two to three servings a week of fish rich in omega-3 EFAs, such as salmon, mackerel, herring, and sardines. These substances have been shown to reduce inflammation in the body and may help ease aches and pains.
- Unless you have respiratory or heart problems, exercise vigorously enough to raise your heart rate a little for at least thirty minutes several days a week. Retaining flexibility really helps the body to stay comfortable and keep moving.
- Do some gentle wake-up stretches in the morning.
- Try taking EPA and DHA (eicosapentaenoic acid and docosahexaenoic acid) and krill oil supplements, which have been shown to alleviate arthritis pain, possibly by helping the body create anti-inflammatory prostaglandins that reduce joint swelling. (Avoid cod liver oil, which contains high levels of vitamins A and D that can be harmful in excess.)
- Glucosamine and chondroitin supplements can also help to relubricate cartilage and regenerate the cushioning in stiff joints.

Lisa's Story

Lisa is a sixty-two-year-old woman who lives in Maryland. She had a number of unwanted postmenopause symptoms and had been diagnosed with osteoporosis.

When I met Maryon I hadn't had a period for four years, but I was still experiencing hot flashes and night sweats. My worst symptoms were insomnia and almost nonexistent sex drive. Even though I have a wonderful and gorgeous husband, I couldn't face sex, as it was so painful due to vaginal dryness. I've had lifelong aches and pains, as I was diagnosed with arthritis when I was fourteen years old. I felt forgetful, overweight, irritable, nervous, bloated to the point of looking six months pregnant, and my skin was uncharacteristically dry.

I didn't have high hopes, as I had tried most things to feel better, but I followed Maryon's tailor-made recommendations completely, as I was so desperate. I thoroughly enjoyed the diet she suggested, took a number of supplements that she thought would help me, and made time for exercise and formal relaxation. Amazingly, within weeks I had no bloating, and my husband's bloating is greatly reduced too, as he's been following my new way of eating.

Even after a month my dry vagina is wet again, and both my husband and I are delighted to say that sex is back on the menu. The hot flashes and night sweats are already greatly reduced, and unbelievably, 80 percent of the joint pain that I have lived with practically my whole life has gone! I'm sleeping better and no longer need a sleeping pill, and if I do wake in the night, I get straight back to sleep now. I've lost weight, I'm able to concentrate and listen, and I am no longer forgetful. This program has truly been a life changer for me.

What the Research Says

Hot flashes are thought to be partly caused by the brain's response to fluctuating hormones. An Italian study suggests that supplementing the diet with omega-3 and omega-6 fatty acids can significantly reduce the number of hot flashes. The randomized, double-blind, placebo-controlled crossover trial found that these supplements led to a significant decrease in severe hot flashes in twenty-nine women over twenty-four weeks. EFAs may help attenuate hormonal ups and downs by acting on nerve membranes and neurotransmitters.

Omega-3 EFAs also have a positive effect on blood triglycerides and HDL, the "good" cholesterol, according to Australian researchers who conducted a randomized, double-blind placebo-controlled trial on fifty-three perimenopausal women who took 1 gram per day of omega-3 EFAs.

Another Italian study of 66,500 women attending menopause clinics showed that those suffering severe hot flashes and night sweats were less active than other participants.

Data from the Melbourne Women's Midlife Health Project traced thirty-five women over eight years. Daily exercisers were less likely to be bothered with hot flashes.

I'm happier, sleeping well, and more contented. I don't lose my memory anymore, I'm very on the ball and young again in my mind.

— Sharyn McLaughlin

Several studies show that isoflavones — naturally occurring estrogen-like substances found in soy and some other plants — help reduce hot flashes and night sweats, improve cognitive function and memory, and lessen the appearance of wrinkles.

Researchers in Turkey studying a group of 303 women found that higher vitamin D levels are associated with fewer menopausal symptoms and better sexual function. They therefore recommend that vitamin D status should be evaluated in all menopausal women.

Following a healthy lifestyle and finding time to relax also seems to help with hot flashes and night sweats. Consuming a diet rich in isoflavones (see page 60) and omega-3 and omega-6 oils, getting regular exercise, cutting down on alcohol, and taking time to relax can all help alleviate these symptoms.

Your Menopause Cheat Sheet

The table below offers a quick guide to remedies for troubling menopause symptoms. You can use it now to get a flying start on your personal Six-Week Natural Menopause Solution, but don't stop here! The following chapters offer in-depth explanations of how these approaches, used in combination, can help you eliminate your symptoms in the long term and feel better than ever.

Since many symptoms can be relieved by simple dietary changes, I suggest you also refer to the list of nutritional content of foods (page 222) and the meal plans in chapter 11 to identify nutritious foods and easy ways to incorporate them into your diet.

Symptoms	Possible Causes	How To Feel Better
Hot flashes and night sweats	Deficiencies of estrogen, magnesium, calcium, and vitamin D	Eat plenty of foods that contain naturally occurring phytoestrogens, such as soy-based products and flaxseed. Take red clover supplements. Consider taking magnesium, calcium, and vitamin D supplements. Avoid hot drinks, spicy foods, alcohol, and caffeine, which can increase your body temperature and trigger these symptoms.
Headaches and migraines	Deficiencies of vitamin E, B vitamins, and magnesium	Eat regular, wholesome meals and snacks to keep blood sugar in check. Avoid caffeine. Take a multivitamin and a magnesium supplement. Try incorporating ginger into your diet; it is a known relaxant and has anti-inflammatory properties that can ease headaches.
Vaginal dryness and loss of libido	Deficiencies of estrogen, essential fatty acids, vitamins D and E, zinc, and magnesium	Eat plant-based foods that contain phytoestrogens. Consider taking sea buckthorn oil, vitamins D and E, zinc, and magnesium supplements.
Mood swings and depression	Deficiencies of vitamins B1, B3, B6, B12, C, and D; folate; biotin; and possibly essential fatty acids	Avoid processed foods, which are low in nutrients. Include plenty of greens, nuts, seeds, and berries in your diet. Exercise regularly. Consider taking supplements of vitamin B complex, vitamins C and D, and fish oils.

Symptoms	Possible Causes	How To Feel Better
Insomnia	Deficiency of B vitamins (in particular vitamin B12), magnesium, and calcium	Avoid caffeine. Eat lean meat and seafood, which contain B vitamins. Avoid going hungry, to keep blood sugar from dropping. Take B vitamins, calcium, and magnesium supplements.
Panic attacks and palpitations	Deficiencies of potassium, magnesium, and iron	Avoid caffeine. Eat potassium-rich foods, like bananas. Consider taking iron and magnesium supplements, as well as herbs including maca, valerian, or St. John's wort.
Joint and muscle aches	Deficiencies of magnesium, potassium, sodium, vitamin B1, and vitamin D	Consume 2–3 servings of omega-3-rich fish per week. Eat bananas. Consider taking vitamin D and omega-3 supplements.
Fatigue	Deficiencies of protein, iron, magnesium, potassium, B vitamins, and vitamins C and D	Eat unprocessed foods. Include nuts, seeds, omega-3-rich fish, and fresh fruit and vegetables in your regular diet. Consume plenty of protein. Consider taking a multivitamin and supplementing with vitamins C and D and magnesium.
Memory loss and poor concentration	Deficiencies of iron, vitamins B1, B12, and D, folate, and possibly essential fatty acids	Eat wholesome foods that include soy. Consider taking multivitamins and supplements containing minerals, vitamin D, and fish oils.

Symptoms	Possible Causes	How To Feel Better
Thinning hair	Deficiencies of estrogen, iron, and vitamin C	Eat a phytoestrogen-rich diet. Get your iron levels checked and take a supplement if necessary. Consider taking a multivitamin and additional vitamin C.
Restless legs	Deficiencies of iron and folate	Avoid caffeine. Get your iron and folate levels checked and take supplements if necessary.

Chapter 2

WEEK TWO

Diet and Hormones

So far, looking at what's happening in the body at midlife, we've seen that many symptoms can be explained by the natural drop in our estrogen levels. However, that's not usually the whole story: there may be other underlying causes. Diet and lifestyle play an important part in the experience of menopause as well as in our general health and well-being. You've probably heard the adage "You are what you eat," and to a large degree it's true. Mother Nature has provided us with many sources of goodies: we just have to know what to eat at each life stage to protect and enhance our health. In this chapter we explore the link between diet and hormones and the nutritional deficiencies that aggravate symptoms of menopause.

Menopause is often a time when nutritional deficiencies start to become apparent. Years of wear and tear, pregnancy, and breastfeeding can all challenge our nutrient stores. If we don't know how to replace what time and nature have taken away, we may be left in a nutritionally depleted state, which can affect our brain chemistry and our hormone balance.

You may think your diet is healthy, but if you start to analyze it more closely, a different story might emerge. A few years ago, a group of staff at a magazine company in the UK completed questionnaires for me about their diet and nutritional health. Not one of the participants was consuming an adequate diet, and all had some signs of nutritional deficiencies. Most of us lack knowledge about how to meet all our body's nutritional needs.

Changing Times

Today's diet is very different from that of our Stone Age ancestors. Three million years ago, vegetable matter, including hard seeds and plant fiber such as roots and stems, was the mainstay of our diet, rather than the large amounts of animal protein many people consume today. And the meat produced by intensive farming is much higher in fat, especially saturated fat, than the wild meat eaten by our ancestors.

Our lifestyle is also very different even from that of just seventy-five years ago, when three balanced meals, with just the occasional between-meal snack, were the norm. Today, many of us struggle to eat one or two balanced meals a day, with several snacks. We often eat convenience food and commercially prepared meals on the run, rather than the wholesome, home-cooked foods favored by many of our grandmothers.

Add to this the fact that we exercise much less than we used to, and it's not surprising that we suffer from conditions such as heart disease, cancer, diabetes, and osteoporosis to a far greater degree than people did even a few decades ago. The incidence of conditions such as irritable bowel syndrome, constipation, diarrhea with painful gas, bloating, migraine headaches, nervous tension, irritability, insomnia, and feelings of aggression and fatigue are also on the rise.

Are You Fit for Midlife? Results from a Survey

My team and I conducted an online survey of more than 1,200 women between the ages of thirty-five and sixty-four to assess their health prospects for midlife. We found that lifestyle factors such as poor diet, lack of exercise, alcohol intake, and smoking seemed to be strongly linked with mental and physical health problems. Only a quarter of the women in the survey were achieving the following five targets for a healthy midlife:

- Eating two 4-ounce servings of fish a week, including at least one serving of oily fish
- Eating five servings of fruit and vegetables a day
- Exercising at least five times a week
- Consuming no more than seven large glasses of alcohol a week
- Not smoking

In addition, almost 50 percent of respondents said they did not feel as healthy as they used to. Seventeen percent smoked more than ten cigarettes a day, and 8 percent smoked between one and ten cigarettes a day.

On a more positive note, 75 percent of the women said they would be willing to modify their diet. A similar percentage said they would be willing to do more exercise. Fifty-five percent said they would consider taking supplements, and 40 percent were willing to incorporate relaxation into their timetable.

Interestingly, respondents who were achieving all five targets reported much higher libido than the others in the group. Their energy levels and their general sense of well-being were noticeably better too.

Hormones in the Balance

What we eat influences our health and hormone function. In particular, hormonal balance can be affected by the amount of fat and fiber in our diet, as well as by levels of individual essential nutrients.

Although we still don't fully understand the relative importance of these factors, it is safe to say that they have been largely overlooked in the treatment of midlife symptoms, even though research now shows that billions of women around the world have nutritional deficiencies. Dietary changes offer one alternative to hormone therapy for the control of estrogen withdrawal symptoms. A change of diet may also help lower the risk of heart disease and hormone-related cancers of the breast and uterus.

Scientific interest in the effect of dietary fat on health originally arose because of the strong links between fat consumption and both heart disease and breast cancer. Women in countries where the diet is typically high in fat, especially the saturated fat found mainly in animal products, have high rates of breast cancer. We don't yet know whether reducing animal fat intake reduces the risk of breast cancer, but we do know that the fat and fiber content of our diet can affect hormone function. Fiber binds to estrogen in the small intestine, helping to balance our hormone levels.

A diet high in animal fat and low in fiber is associated with relatively high levels of circulating estrogen. The US Food and Nutrition Board of the National Institute of Medicine recommends that women under fifty consume 25 grams of dietary fiber per day, while those over fifty should consume 21 grams (to correspond with an overall reduction in food intake for older women). Most Americans, however, get only 15 grams per day. It may be that Western women who have followed high-fat, low-fiber diets are more likely to experience estrogen withdrawal symptoms at midlife because their bodies are used to a relatively high level of estrogen. As a result, they don't tolerate the natural drop in estrogen at menopause as well as women who have lower levels of circulating estrogen.

In theory, this means that making a dramatic change to a low-fat, high-fiber diet could aggravate symptoms of estrogen withdrawal in some women. This effect is likely to be offset by the fact that the diet is healthier, which in turn has a positive effect on hormone function. But if you do change your diet at the time of menopause, it makes sense to do so gradually. For example, don't suddenly go from being a meat eater to following a weight-loss vegan diet. You need to give your body time to adjust.

Essential Nutrients

Our body requires many nutrients in order to produce hormones and enable them to do their job properly. Severe nutritional deficiencies are rare in countries like the United States, Canada, Australia, and the United Kingdom, but our surveys suggest that many women in these countries have chronic deficiencies of essential nutrients, beginning well before menopause. For example, 50 to 80 percent of women with PMS have low levels of magnesium, B vitamins, vitamin D, zinc, iron, calcium, and EFAs. Low levels of important nutrients leave women in what I call "economy mode." Below I discuss some essential nutrients and their function. Foods rich in these nutrients are included in the list beginning on page 222.

Iron

Iron is essential to the production of hemoglobin, the compound in our red blood cells that transports oxygen from our lungs to all the cells in the body. The muscles and brain also need iron, and it is a vital component of many of the enzymes that drive the chemical reactions in our cells. Low levels of iron can lead to brittle and split nails, hair loss, and anemia, which can cause fatigue. Around 4 percent of women of childbearing age are anemic; severe anemia can cause periods to stop. An additional 10 percent of menstruating women suffer from a mild iron deficiency. Heavier periods, common in perimenopause, can further deplete iron levels.

B Vitamins

Broadly speaking, B vitamins are involved in releasing energy from food. A severe deficiency in vitamin B12 can cause periods to become irregular, a symptom that may be confused with perimenopause among women in their early forties. A lack of vitamin B12, which is found in red meat and other foods, can occur in vegans and in older people who lose the ability to absorb this vitamin. Symptoms include weight loss, fatigue, tingling in the feet, and balance problems.

Vitamin B6 deficiency, which is often linked with premenstrual syndrome, is surprisingly common, and it is associated with anxiety and depression in both men and women. It is involved in the response of tissues to estrogen and seems to be needed by the part of a cell's surface that interacts with estrogen receptors. So increased amounts of vitamin B6 may be necessary if you take relatively large amounts of estrogen — for example if you take oral contraceptives.

Vitamin B1 deficiency is also associated with anxiety and depression.

A lack of vitamin B3 (niacin, nicotinic acid, or niacinamide) usually develops only in heavy drinkers, those on very poor, low-protein diets, and those with serious digestive problems. Symptoms include depression, diarrhea, and a red, scaly rash on the face, the back of the hands, or other areas exposed to light. In women who are deficient in vitamin B3, menstrual irregularities are common, and this deficiency may aggravate symptoms in perimenopausal women who drink heavily.

Vitamin D

Vitamin D deficiency is now known to have many serious health implications. Dietary sources of vitamin D include egg yolks, fortified milk and cereals, cheese, and oily fish. The vitamin can also be synthesized in our skin from sunlight, but people who spend most of their time indoors, and those who always cover or protect their skin while outdoors, rarely receive enough sun exposure to maintain healthy levels of vitamin D — particularly in the winter, when days are shorter and sunlight is weaker. US health guidelines recommend taking a vitamin D3 supplement of 600 international units (IU) daily in the winter. Those who are housebound or always cover their skin should take vitamin D throughout the year.

Vitamin D plays a role in calcium metabolism, so it is crucial to bone growth and health, helping to prevent the bone-thinning disease osteoporosis. There is also mounting evidence that low levels of vitamin D are associated with an increased risk of type 1 diabetes, bone and muscle pain, hypertension, and cancers of the breast, ovaries, colon, esophagus, lymphatic system, and prostate.

Symptoms of deficiency include excessive sweating — which is obviously a key issue for women already suffering from hot flashes at midlife — along with low mood, aching joints, muscles and bones, and recurrent urinary tract infections, all common symptoms as we age.

During the summer at most latitudes, about twenty minutes' exposure of the face and arms a day, early in the day or evening, without heavy sunscreen, should provide you with enough vitamin D for the health of your bones. If you have fair skin, it's probably best to restrict exposure to sunlight to ten minutes without sunscreen. The ultraviolet radiation that damages our skin is strongest between 10 a.m. and 4 p.m. If you have to go outdoors during the middle of the day, be sure to protect your skin from damage and signs of aging with a good sunscreen.

Vitamin E

Scientists discovered long ago that a deficiency of vitamin E in rats caused pregnant females to lose their offspring. In fact, the chemical name for vitamin E is tocopherol, which is derived from the Greek words for "childbearing." Vitamin E is an antioxidant, helping to repair the effects of free radicals (unstable chemical molecules that can damage cells). It is also thought to help reduce inflammation.

In women with premenstrual syndrome, supplements of vitamin E have been found to raise estrogen levels, but its effect on hormone chemistry in perimenopausal and postmenopausal women has not been studied to any great degree. Its effect on hot flashes, however, has been known since 1949. In one of the first studies, a positive response, with over 50 percent fewer hot flashes, was recorded when high doses were given (in the region of 1,000 IU per day), although this small, early trial was not sufficiently robust to convince today's doctors.

Low vitamin E levels have been associated with an elevated risk of breast cancer, so supplementation might help some women, perhaps those in perimenopause rather than those who are postmenopausal.

Good sources of vitamin E include almonds, hazelnuts, Brazil and pine nuts, sweet potato, and sunflower and rapeseed oils.

Magnesium

Magnesium is necessary for normal bone, muscle, and nerve function and for the production of energy in cells. Like potassium, it controls energy functions within cells. Good sources include fresh fruit and vegetables, especially green ones. But magnesium deficiency is common: the National Health and Nutrition Examination Survey (NHANES) of 2013–16 found that 48 percent of Americans ingest less magnesium from food and beverages than the estimated average requirement for their age group.

Magnesium is also involved in reproductive hormone function. Experiments have shown that the ovaries need it to respond to the stimulatory effect of the pituitary hormones FSH and LH. A failure by the ovaries to respond is exactly what happens at menopause. Since magnesium supplementation can reduce PMS symptoms, it's not surprising that it has also been shown to alleviate some menopausal problems, including mood swings, anxiety, insomnia, and bladder problems.

Women experiencing an early menopause, erratic menstrual cycles, fatigue, anxiety, depression, or aches and pains may benefit from magnesium supplementation. A diet naturally high in magnesium is also rich in other nutrients, and supplements are harmless enough. The only likely side effect is diarrhea, and the laxative effect could actually help if you are constipated.

At last studies are beginning to look at the relationship between magnesium and the timing of menopausal symptoms. This is great news, because magnesium levels are known to be low in at least 50 percent of women with PMS and in some women with menopausal problems.

Zinc

Only 0.003 percent of our body is made up of zinc, but without it we wouldn't be able to live. The average intake of zinc has decreased over the last sixty years (to below World War II levels in the United Kingdom), mainly because we now eat less red meat. Zinc intake in many Western countries, including the US, the UK, and Australia, is fairly close to the minimum recommended amounts. In addition, absorption of zinc is reduced by consumption of alcohol, whole grains, and many other foods.

Zinc is involved in a wide range of metabolic processes. More than 85 percent of our total body zinc is found in our muscles and bones. We require it to make insulin, for the catalytic activity of about one hundred enzymes, and for normal mental, immune system, and sex hormone function. It is also involved in the absorption of other key nutrients.

The best dietary source of zinc is oysters, followed by beef and most other meats. Vegetarian sources include Brazil nuts, almonds, muesli, lentils, and eggs.

Calcium

Calcium intake is important in the prevention of osteoporosis, but that is only part of the story. On average we carry approximately three pounds (1.4 kg) of calcium in our bodies, 99 percent of it in our bones and the rest circulating in our bloodstream. Blood calcium is necessary for blood clotting, optimum muscle and cardiac function, and neurotransmission.

Calcium is essential for growing strong bones in children, but it's also important as we age. If we consume insufficient calcium throughout our lives, we may approach middle and old age with a low bone mass and a high risk of osteoporosis. In addition, because calcium in the bloodstream is vital to bodily functions, if blood calcium becomes low, it is leached from our bones into the bloodstream.

The average calcium intake in the US for women is generally lower than the recommended daily intake, which ranges from 1,000 mg for women in their forties to 1,200 mg for those age fifty and over. While the minimum amount of calcium required daily is a controversial issue, the World Health Organization sets it at 500 mg. Some of the richest sources of calcium are sardines and other small, bony fish, Cheddar cheese, soy, Brazil nuts, spinach, and milk.

Up to two-thirds of our calcium intake may never reach our bones. Other nutrients, including vitamins D and K2 and the minerals magnesium and zinc, are necessary for optimum calcium absorption. Common foods such as whole grains, legumes, and tea are rich in phytates (phytic acid), which can interfere with the absorption of calcium. Paradoxically, however, soy products, which are also rich in phytates, appear to reduce the risk of bone loss. A diet rich in salt and animal protein appears to increase calcium excretion in urine.

Women need at least 700 mg of dietary calcium each day. To assess how much calcium you are getting in your diet, you can use the International Osteoporosis Foundation calculator at www.iofbonehealth.org/calcium-calculator.

Potassium

Potassium is an essential mineral that has many important functions and benefits, including regulating blood pressure, nervous system function, and our body's fluid balance; helping to maintain strong bones; and decreasing the risk of stroke and kidney stones. It is referred to as an electrolyte, because when it's dissolved in water it produces positively charged ions, which are important for many biochemical processes in our body. Rich sources of potassium include fruit, especially bananas; vegetables, including leafy greens, mushrooms, and avocado; and fish, particularly salmon. Different health agencies have different recommendations for intake. According to WHO, we need 3,510 mg per day. NHANES (the US National Health and Nutrition Examination Survey), recommends 4,700 mg per day but reports that fewer than 2 percent of American adults achieve this.

Essential Fatty Acids

Although we are often advised to reduce consumption of fats, not all fats are equal. Some types of fats are essential to our bodily functions. Fats provide us with twice the energy of carbohydrates or sugar. Let's take a look at the various kinds of dietary fats.

The majority of animal fats and some oils from tropical plants are saturated (with hydrogen molecules). These fats are usually solid at room temperature. They provide calories but few other nutritional benefits, and they can contribute to high levels of LDL ("bad") cholesterol in the blood. A diet rich in these saturated animal fats, and lacking in fiber, vitamins, and minerals is considered a risk factor for heart disease.

Many but not all vegetable fats are polyunsaturated. These fats, which are usually liquid at room temperature, do not increase the risk of heart disease in the way that saturated fats do. The same is true of olive and rapeseed oil, which are monounsaturated fats.

Within the polyunsaturated fats is a special category, known as essential fatty acids, or EFAs, which have a number of important functions in the body, including regulating nervous system and hormone function and building cell membranes. Signs of EFA deficiency include dry skin, lifeless hair, cracked nails, fatigue, depression, dry eyes, lack of motivation, aching joints, difficulty in losing weight, forgetfulness, and breast pain — all common symptoms during menopause. If you have tried to lose weight by going on a low-fat or no-fat diet, you are likely to be deficient in EFAs.

On the hormone front, EFAs do something very interesting. They are used in the building of cell walls and, in particular, seem to influence the function of the pieces of cell machinery that are embedded in cell walls, such as hormone receptors. So it is possible that a long-term deficiency of EFAs might modify the way the body responds to certain hormones.

Because our bodies cannot produce EFAs, we must obtain them from food or supplements. Good sources of essential fatty acids are corn, sunflower, and safflower oils, which contain what are known as omega-6 EFAs. Oily fish such as mackerel, herring, and salmon, together with soybean, walnut, and, to a lesser degree, rapeseed oil, contain omega-3 EFAs.

Certain preparations of EFAs have been shown to be beneficial for a variety of conditions. Evening primrose oil contains omega-6 EFAs, which can help women with premenstrual breast tenderness and also some adults and children with eczema. Fish oils have also been shown to reduce the pain and inflammation of rheumatoid arthritis and to lower the levels of some blood fats, though not cholesterol.

According to our midlife survey, those regularly consuming a diet rich in omega-3 EFAs had fewer aches and pains, fewer mood swings, less depression, far more energy, and increased libido.

Making your diet more nutrient dense can only help your hormones to function normally. Take a look at the list of the nutritional content of foods on page 222 to choose nutrient-rich foods you enjoy.

Anne's Story

Anne was a single mother, age fifty-three, when she joined my Facebook group. She felt like a shadow of her former self both physically and mentally.

It started around the age of forty-seven. I had bad heart palpitations, especially in the night. I was in the third year of my degree, so I put it down to stress, but then it continued well after graduation, and I started to get very bad anxiety about even the smallest thing. I felt so stressed, as I would catastrophize about things. I gained weight, I got terrible aches and pains, and I couldn't even dress myself properly. I then developed very vicious migraine attacks and thought I had early-onset dementia, as I lost my concentration. I was forgetting things and doing crazy things like putting my mobile phone in the refrigerator.

Then one night I was driving back from a trip with my son, and, although I was on a familiar road that I had driven on for years, I didn't know where I was, which was terrifying. Plus, I was dealing with a teenager whose hormones were raging at the same time as mine. We argued so often, I was afraid I would lose him as he would go to live with his father.

I went to see my doctor, and he gave me antidepressants, but they just caused side effects. I went in to see another female doctor, completely sobbing, and was told it was part of the aging process.

I was struggling at work, as I had issues with productivity due to lack of concentration. I was tired all the time. I felt like I was under a heavy cloak of fatigue, and my creativity had long since left the building. I couldn't organize my thoughts, which was very scary, and I was desperate for help.

Only weeks after I began Maryon's program, I noticed a huge difference. My energy began to return, and the migraines lessened. As I progressed, my concentration returned, the headaches went completely, and I had an incredible amount of energy. I remember during the fifth week of the course, I got up on a sunny morning and woke my son up and told him we were going on a hike. I made a packed lunch, and we went on a ten-mile adventure and took lots of gorgeous pictures. I will never forget my son saying, "Mum, it's so nice to have you back."

It's been a year now since I undertook Maryon's program, and I really feel better than I can remember. Instead of contemplating leaving the workplace, as I felt unable to function at work, I am now doing so well I have been offered and taken promotion. I'm beyond delighted on so many levels.

Are You Nutritionally Healthy?

Common deficiencies of nutrients like iron, zinc, calcium, magnesium, some B vitamins, and vitamin D affect how we look and feel. Facial acne, greasy skin, cracking at the corners of the mouth, red patches at the sides of the nose, acne on the upper arms or thighs, unmanageable hair, and split, brittle nails can be our body's ways of saying that all is not well — but many of us may not be tuned in to the communication. So let's try to interpret what your body may be trying to tell you.

Refer to the picture on the next page, and then be brave and have a close look in the mirror. Use use the first column of the table on pages 50–54 to check off any signs you notice. You may be surprised at how many of these signs you see in yourself. Some of them may be associated with chronic health conditions that you're already managing; if that's the case, it may be harder to alleviate the problems, but keep in mind that good nutrition can only help.

Realizing that you may be short of certain nutrients is the first step. The next step is putting it right. It's not just a question of taking a supplement, but also of examining your diet and lifestyle, and learning which habits may interfere with your absorption of good nutrients. Binge eating, drinking too much alcohol, and living life in the fast lane take their toll not only on how you feel but also on your appearance.

Manifestations of Nutritional Deficiencies

Wrinkles: antioxidants, selenium, vitamins A, C, and E

Psoriasis: folic acid, zinc, selenium, calcium, omega-3 EFAs

Cracking at corners of eyes: vitamins B2 and B6

Red, greasy skin at sides of nose: vitamins B2 and B6, zinc

Pale complexion: iron, vitamin B12, folic acid

Cracking at corners of mouth: iron, vitamins B2 and B6

Sore, smooth tongue or recurrent mouth ulcers: iron, folic acid, vitamins B12 and B3

Dandruff: biotin, omega-3 EFAs

Generalized hair loss: iron, vitamin C

Eczema: zinc, B vitamins, omega-6 EFAs

Poor night vision: vitamin A, zinc

Red, scaly skin rash: vitamin B3

Dry skin: vitamins A and E

Cracking, peeling skin on lips: vitamin B12

Red tongue tip: vitamins B2 and B6

Soft, bleeding, spongy gums: vitamin C

Brittle nails or flattened, upturned nails: iron

Skin and Hair Problems		
✔ Sign or Symptom	**Possible Causes**	**Solution**
Excessively dry skin	Mixed deficiency of EFAs, vitamin A, and vitamin E	Multivitamin and mineral supplement with evening primrose oil and high-strength fish oil and 400 IU of vitamin E per day
Wrinkles	Deficiencies of antioxidants (vitamins A, C, E, selenium, and zinc)	Strong multivitamin and mineral supplement and soy-rich supplements (see page 63)
Cracking at the corners of the mouth	Iron deficiency B vitamin deficiencies Thrush (Candida) infection	Multivitamin with iron See your doctor if problem persists.
Excessive peeling and cracking of lips	Vitamin B12 deficiency	Vitamin B complex supplement
Red, oily skin at the sides of the nose	Vitamin B2 deficiency Vitamin B6 deficiency Zinc deficiency	Vitamin B complex supplement and 15 mg zinc per day
Combination oily-dry skin	B vitamin deficiencies Zinc deficiency	Vitamin B complex supplement and 15 mg zinc per day
Persistent dandruff	Biotin deficiency EFA deficiencies	Multivitamin, 500 mcg biotin, and high-strength fish oil supplement Antifungal, tea tree, or tar-based shampoo
Excessive skin itching	Deficiencies of vitamins A, B, C, and D	Strong multivitamin and mineral supplement

	Skin and Hair Problems		
✔	**Sign or Symptom**	**Possible Causes**	**Solution**
	Eczema (dry, itchy, reddened skin)	Omega-6 EFA deficiency	Evening primrose oil 3,000 mg per day See your doctor for allergy and infection assessment.
	Red, scaly skin in sun-exposed areas	Vitamin B3 deficiency	Vitamin B complex supplement containing 100 mg of vitamin B3
	Psoriasis	Possible mixed vitamin B, zinc, and EFA deficiencies	Multivitamin, 15 mg zinc per day, and high-strength fish oil supplement combined with conventional medical treatment
	Acne	Zinc deficiency	15 mg zinc per day (30 mg if under medical supervision)
	Rough, red, pimply skin on upper arms or thighs	If severe, mixed vitamin and essential fatty acid deficiencies	Multivitamin and mineral supplement Evening primrose oil 2,000 mg High-strength fish oil Nutritionally dense diet
	Poor hair growth, thinning hair, hair loss	Mild iron deficiency Vitamin C deficiency	Iron and multivitamin supplements 1,000 mg of vitamin C per day See your doctor for specific tests.

Other Symptoms		
✔ **Sign or Symptom**	**Possible Causes**	**Solution**
Food cravings	Chromium deficiency	Chromium supplement 100–200 mcg per day
Fatigue	Anemia B vitamin deficiencies Magnesium deficiency Underactive thyroid	Multivitamin and mineral supplement See your doctor for appropriate blood tests (including vitamin B12 level).
Pale appearance	Anemia Iron or folate deficiency Vitamin B12 deficiency	See your doctor for appropriate blood tests (including vitamin B12 level).
Recurrent mouth ulcers	Iron or folate deficiency Vitamin B12 deficiency	See your doctor for appropriate blood tests (including vitamin B12 level). Multivitamin and iron supplement
Sore, bleeding gums	Vitamin C deficiency	1,000 mg vitamin C with bioflavonoids per day Visit your dental hygienist.
Depression, low mood, low libido, anxiety, PMS	Mixed deficiency of B vitamins, vitamin D, magnesium, and essential fatty acids	Magnesium supplement or Multivitamin and mineral supplement with additional magnesium 150–300 mg per day Strong fish oil supplement Consume oily fish.

Other Symptoms		
✔	**Sign or Symptom**	**Possible Causes**	**Solution**

✔	Sign or Symptom	Possible Causes	Solution
	Split, brittle, flattened, or upturned nails	Iron deficiency	Iron supplement See your doctor if problem persists.
	Ridged nails, white spots on nails	Iron deficiency Zinc deficiency	Multivitamin and mineral supplement Nutritionally dense diet
	Loss of sense of taste	Zinc deficiency	15 mg zinc per day (30 mg if under medical supervision) See your doctor if problem persists.
	Poor appetite	Zinc deficiency Iron deficiency B vitamin deficiencies	Multivitamin and multimineral supplement See your doctor about any significant, unexplained weight loss.
	Poor night vision	Vitamin A (retinol) deficiency Zinc deficiency	Multivitamin 15 mg zinc per day (30 mg if under medical supervision) See your doctor if problem persists.
	Aching joints Muscle pain and cramps	Deficiencies of magnesium, potassium, sodium, vitamin B1, vitamin D, and calcium	Strong multivitamin and mineral supplement Calcium supplement Magnesium supplement Vitamin D supplement

Other Symptoms		
✔ **Sign or Symptom**	**Possible Causes**	**Solution**
Palpitations	Potassium deficiency Magnesium deficiency Anemia	Magnesium supplement Reduce dietary sodium. Consume potassium-rich foods. See your doctor for cardiac function tests.
Restless legs	Iron deficiency Folate deficiency	Iron and folate supplements Consume foods rich in iron and folates.
Numbness and tingling in hands, arms, or feet	B vitamin deficiencies Folate deficiency Essential fatty acids deficiency	Consume foods rich in vitamin B and folates. Consume oily fish. Vitamin, folate, and fish-oil supplements
Painful periods	Magnesium deficiency	150–300 mg magnesium per day Evening primrose oil supplement Fish oil supplement
Irregular periods	Underweight Low-protein diet Excessive alcohol consumption	Strong multivitamin preparation Nutritionally dense diet.
Excessive sweating	Lack of estrogen Vitamin D deficiency	Vitamin D supplement

If you didn't check any of these symptoms, you're a star! You are probably in good nutritional shape and don't need to change your diet or take nutritional supplements, unless you want to take a multivitamin and mineral supplement (see page 82) to protect yourself against the potentially harmful effects of our modern environment.

If you checked more than eight to twelve items, you're not doing too badly, but there are some issues you need to address. Try making your diet more nutrient dense and consider taking the supplements recommended for your particular problems (see page 82).

If you checked more than twelve items, you need to make some fairly major changes to your diet. Read through the meal plans in chapter 11 and consider taking the recommended supplements to address your particular symptoms.

Make a note of any possible deficiencies in your Natural Menopause Solution worksheet (page 232). You can repeat this test in three months' time and compare your scores.

Gail's Story

Gail is a publicist from Los Angeles who was fifty-two when she was referred to me by a mutual contact.

I was scared by the panic attacks, headaches, and dizziness I was experiencing, which resulted in my going to the hospital. The hot flashes, which seemed to come out of nowhere, made me feel even more panic-stricken. I didn't feel able to look after my clients or keep up with my demanding work life, and I had no energy to deal with my family at either end of my working day. I was so exhausted by my lack of good sleep, I'd fall asleep by 9 p.m. after my girls went to bed and then be awake by 2 a.m. with hot flashes. Sex was off the menu, as I felt so awful. In truth, I was like a shadow of my former dynamic self.

I was grateful to be introduced to Maryon, as I was afraid of what the future might hold. I followed the recommendations as closely as I could and within a matter of weeks began to feel so much better. I made time for myself, adjusted my diet, and began exercising and practicing formal relaxation as well as taking the supplements Maryon recommended for me. The headaches went completely. I began sleeping better. The hot flashes and night sweats subsided, and so did the anxiety. I really never thought I would find the old me again, but I am so relieved and grateful that I have. I can think clearly now, work in my usual efficient way, and be there for my family with energy and enthusiasm rather than hiding my overwhelmed self away.

Boosting Your Nutrient Levels

You may have heard the saying that one man's meat is another man's poison. The same is true for diet. Just because a food is deemed healthy doesn't necessarily mean it's going to be great for *you* — at least in the short term. When women have low levels of nutrients, their tolerance for certain foods may be temporarily reduced. If you experience bloating and gas, it may be a good idea to avoid grains initially, including wheat, barley, rye, and maybe even oats — including bran from these grains.

In the next chapter I focus on Mother Nature's estrogen and how you can beat bloating and curb cravings.

Since embarking on Maryon's program I feel like a completely different person. It's like someone pressed the reset button and I'm once again the person I was! My husband completely agrees.

— Lilly Roads

Chapter 3

WEEK THREE

Replacing Estrogen Naturally

What if I told you that Mother Nature could outsmart your brain, fooling it into believing that you once again had normal levels of estrogen circulating in your body and eliminating or reducing symptoms of menopause? I teach women how to do this every day.

At menopause our ovaries are no longer serving us with regular amounts of estrogen. The estrogen receptors in our cells signal this lack. Our brain doesn't know what's going on, so it attempts to kick-start the ovaries back into function by sending thermal surges through our body that we call hot flashes and night sweats. What can we do to reduce them? Besides bringing nutrients back into an optimum range, which has a normalizing effect on brain chemistry and hormones, my Six-Week Natural Menopause Solution is also designed to provide small amounts of phytoestrogens — estrogen-like compounds from plants — throughout the day. By binding to the estrogen receptors in our cells, these compounds fool the brain into believing there is a significant amount of estrogen circulating in the body.

Although phytoestrogens are only about one-thousandth as potent as the estrogen produced by the body, they have been hailed by many as the natural alternative to hormone replacement therapy HRT. These neat little substances can not only soothe menopausal symptoms but also protect us against heart disease, dementia, and osteoporosis. They may also help lower the risk of hormone-related cancers in both women and men (some types of breast, ovarian, and prostate cancer).

Benefits of Phytoestrogens

- Reduce menopausal hot flashes
- Prevent bone loss
- Reduce blood levels of LDL ("bad") cholesterol and raise HDL ("good") cholesterol
- Unblock clogged arteries
- Normalize blood glucose levels
- Regulate the menstrual cycle
- Help prevent estrogen-related cancers
- Improve cognitive function
- Restore memory

How Do Phytoestrogens Work?

A wealth of research has shown that a regular intake of phytoestrogens throughout the day can play a useful part in controlling menopause symptoms, producing effects similar to treatment with HRT. Two kinds of phytoestrogen have been found to be particularly effective: isoflavones, derived from soy products and red clover, and lignans, found in flaxseeds (also known as linseeds).

Isoflavones are fast becoming known as great hormone regulators, as they help to keep estrogen circulating in our system. When estrogen is in oversupply in the body, as can happen before menopause, isoflavones play musical chairs with estrogen, competing for the receptor sites in cells. (Receptors are structures found on the surface of cells that allow specific hormones and other chemicals into cells, rather like a key in a lock.) Some of the isoflavones displace the body's own estrogen and, being weaker, may mitigate estrogen's cancer-promoting effects.

As estrogen levels start to drop around the time of menopause, isoflavones have the opposite effect, binding to estrogen receptors in the absence of estrogen. Combined with supplements and regular relaxation, consuming isoflavones can help ease hot flashes and night sweats. In Asia, where the typical diet is high in isoflavones, women over the age of forty-five rarely experience menopausal symptoms such as hot flashes and night sweats. In fact, the term *hot flash* had no equivalent in the Japanese language until recently. An isoflavone-rich diet can also protect against osteoporosis, memory loss, and heart disease in the long-term.

Merle's Story

Merle is a jewelry designer from Sydney, Australia. Her symptoms were over-shadowing her life, and she consulted me when sleep deprivation started to get the better of her and inhibited her daily functioning.

My worst symptoms were the regular and intense hot flashes, resulting in an overwhelming sense of lethargy. It turned me into a stranger, and even my family said I had such a poor quality of life that it needed to be addressed. I was delighted to discover that there was a solution to my troubles. Recommendations included making dietary changes, taking supplements, exercise, and relaxation.

Even though I'm not really a pill person, I took the supplements Maryon recommended for me and found that the benefits far outweighed any misgivings I had. Within a month, I noticed the intensity of my symptoms had reduced. Over the next month, the flashes almost completely disappeared, and I got my energy back. I went from having no real quality of life to feeling absolutely excellent!

Putting Phytoestrogens on the Menu

If you're concerned that including isoflavones calls for a radical change of diet, don't worry. There are so many delicious options to choose from that you'll soon find ways to incorporate them into your daily routine. And you don't have to become vegetarian overnight either. To alleviate menopausal symptoms, you should consume 100 mg of isoflavones each day. (The amount in a typical Western diet is about 3 mg.) Working out the exact amount can be tricky because, unlike supplements, foods don't contain standardized amounts, and isoflavones appear to leave the body quite quickly, reaching peak levels in the bloodstream within five or six hours of consumption. The best way to ensure that you get enough is to consume small amounts of phytoestrogen-rich foods often throughout the day.

The richest food sources of isoflavones are soy products, including soy milk, tofu, edamame beans (immature soybeans in the pod), miso paste, and soy flour. The most lignan-rich food is flaxseed. Smaller quantities of isoflavones are found in lentils, chickpeas, mung and other beans, green and yellow vegetables, and sunflower, pumpkin, and sesame seeds. Additionally, red clover is a rich source, but it must be taken in the form of supplements (see page 82).

Foods rich in phytoestrogen, including ready-made foods for those short of time to cook, are now readily available from most supermarkets and health food stores, and there are many delicious treats you can whip up yourself in minutes. Soy yogurts are widely available, and soy milkshakes make a handy snack. The recipe section beginning on page 187 includes a delicious fruit loaf made with soy and flaxseeds, as well as smoothies, tasty whipped desserts, pancakes, and snack bars, all designed to make soy palatable and enjoyable. The list of phytoestrogen-rich foods below shows the approximate amount of isoflavones per serving. Asterisks indicate recipes provided in chapter 12.

If you consume a phytoestrogen-rich breakfast, such as phyto muesli with soy milk, then have a couple of additional "phyto fixes," such as soy yogurt, a handful of edamame beans, or a slice of soy fruit loaf in the afternoon and evening, you should start to gain control over your hot flashes and other menopausal symptoms.

Isoflavone Content of Foods	
Food (serving size)	Isoflavones (mg)
Tempeh (100 g/3.5 ounces)	60
Canned soybeans (100 g/3.5 ounces)	53
Edamame beans, raw (100 g/3.5 ounces)	40
Raw sprouted soy seeds (100 g/3.5 ounces)	34
Bowl of phyto muesli* with soy milk and flaxseeds	30
Tofu (100 g/3.5 ounces)	25
Soy milk (250 mL/1 cup)	20
Tub of whipped soy dessert	20
Soy fruit shake (250 mL/1 cup)	20
Edamame beans, cooked (100 g/3.5 ounces)	18
Soy yogurt (100 g/3.5 ounces)	17
Soy and linseed bread (1 slice)	11
Slice of phyto fruit loaf*	10
Low-fat soy milk	10
Phyto fix bar*	10
Soy and rice pancakes* (2)	10

Note: Although soy is a great source of isoflavones and many women enjoy it in various forms, some women can't digest it easily and find it causes abdominal bloating and gas. Sometimes it takes a few weeks for the gut to adjust. It's worth trying different types of soy foods and making notes on what works. Adding ginger to warmed soy milk can sometimes make it more digestible. Consuming probiotics with soy can help with the absorption process. Some women who find soy milk difficult to digest can manage edamame beans. But if you are one of the unlucky ones and soy continues to be problematic for your digestive system, it's important to add other sources of isoflavones to your diet.

Are Phytoestrogens Safe?

Every week, dozens of menopausal women ask whether soy is safe, as they have heard or read conflicting reports.

People in Asia have been consuming substantial amounts of isoflavone-rich foods for hundreds of years with no recorded ill effects. In fact, those consuming a traditional Japanese diet have far lower rates of heart disease, osteoporosis, and estrogen-related cancers like breast, ovarian, and prostate cancer. Although studies have shown positive effects from consuming up to 170 mg of isoflavones daily, the long-term effect of high doses has not been studied. The traditional Asian diet delivers 50–100 mg of isoflavones per day. Similar quantities have been found to have therapeutic effects in several clinical trials.

In the West, numerous medical experts, the American Institute for Cancer Research, and the European Food Safety Authority have concluded on the basis of medical research that soy products are safe and can even have a protective effect on health. Women who have had breast cancer and are now going through menopause can absolutely benefit from consuming soy products.

Because isoflavones can affect thyroid function, I am also asked about whether it's safe to consume soy products if you have thyroid problems. There is plenty of evidence to show that it is safe to do so. However, you may have to work with your doctor during your regular check-ups to adjust your medication.

Overall, soy products help us overcome menopause symptoms. An added bonus is that they can help us to maintain our short- and long- term memory and protect us from heart disease and osteoporosis after menopause.

What about Men and Children?

Mainly because estrogen is associated with women, men are often under a misconception that if they consume foods containing naturally occurring estrogen, they will grow breasts. Some people even think it will have an adverse effect on children. But Asian men have consumed significant quantities of isoflavones for centuries without any apparent adverse health effects. In fact, scientists believe that an isoflavone-rich diet may contribute to the low rates of death among Asian men from both prostate cancer and heart disease. Asian children also typically eat phytoestrogens daily without any known adverse health effects. Mark Messina, who has probably been involved in as much research on isoflavones as any other researcher in the world, believes that the earlier the exposure to phytoestrogen-rich foods, the better.

What the Research Says
Phytoestrogens

A host of studies suggest that phytoestrogens may be as powerful as HRT in protecting against osteoporosis, heart disease, and other unwanted symptoms of menopause. A paper by the Women's Health Practice and Research Network of the American College of Clinical Pharmacy reports that phytoestrogens help alleviate menopausal symptoms as well as reducing the risk of both breast cancer and osteoporosis.

As long ago as 1990, a group of Australian doctors studied a group of women who were going through menopause and not taking HRT. The women followed a diet rich in soy products, organic flaxseeds, and red clover extract. Looking at changes in the vaginal wall lining, the researchers demonstrated that it was possible to bring about the same changes in the lining of the vaginal wall with this diet as with HRT. This study demonstrated that phytoestrogens, including soy isoflavones, can reach the same parts of the body as HRT.

Since then there have been many additional positive studies. An analysis of nineteen clinical trials showed that soybean isoflavone supplements can alleviate the frequency and severity of hot flashes in menopause. Taking isoflavones reduced the frequency of hot flashes by 26 percent. The analysis also showed that supplements providing more than 18.8 mg of genistein (thought to be one of the most potent isoflavones) were more than twice as effective at reducing hot flash frequency than lower-concentration genistein supplements. Another recent review also confirms the effectiveness of soy isoflavones in reducing hot flashes.

In addition, a study in the *American Journal of Clinical Nutrition* concluded that soy isoflavones, although not as potent as risedronate (a drug used to strengthen bone), are effective in preserving bone density in postmenopausal women.

Menopause is associated with an increased risk of heart disease. Previous research has shown that isoflavones protect arteries against oxidative damage, an underlying cause of heart disease. Recently, researchers in Brazil gave ninety-six postmenopausal women a dietary questionnaire, assessed physical activity with a pedometer, and examined the women for subclinical heart disease by measuring the thickness of artery walls and looking for atherosclerotic plaques. They found subclinical early heart disease, with no obvious symptoms, in 35 percent of participants. These women were more likely to consume less selenium, magnesium, folate, and isoflavones than the women without heart disease. Having a high body mass index, which often equates to being overweight, was also associated with a 90 percent higher risk of early heart disease. Higher estrogen levels and isoflavone intake were independently associated with a lower risk of heart disease.

Soybean supplements may also help with the depression that plagues so many women at menopause. A pilot study has shown that such supplements enhance the effects of antidepressants. Forty depressed menopausal women were given either antidepressants alone or soybean alone, or antidepressants plus soybean. Women on the combination of medication and soy reported significantly greater improvement in their depression than the other groups. The results suggest that that soybean extracts both have an antidepressant effect in their own right and can also enhance the therapeutic effects of antidepressant drugs.

A study from Italy looked at how two different supplements affected menopause-related anxiety, palpitations, and insomnia. The first supplement (known as Estromineral), taken by three hundred women, consisted of 60 mg isoflavones, plus calcium, vitamin D3, and the probiotic *Bacillus coagulans*. The second supplement (known as Estromineral Serena), which contained the same active ingredients along with magnolia bark extract, was taken by 334 women. Both treatments showed a reduction of symptoms after four, eight, and twelve weeks. The second was more effective for insomnia, irritability, anxiety, depression, and loss of libido.

In another recent study, 262 postmenopausal women received either genistein (54 mg daily) or a placebo for two years. Assessment after one and two years showed that genistein improved the women's quality of life (as measured by health status, life satisfaction, and depression) compared with the placebo. A similar effect was found among a group of middle-aged Japanese women on a low dose (25 mg/day) of the isoflavone aglycone, which significantly alleviated symptoms of depression and insomnia.

The use of isoflavone supplements may also have wider implications for women's mental health. A 2015 review looked at evidence from research covering over one thousand women and found that soy isoflavone supplements seemed to improve overall cognitive function and visual memory in postmenopausal women. The best improvements may occur when supplements are started at an earlier age. Further research will reveal whether these supplements offer long-term protection against dementia.

Taking isoflavone supplements can also benefit the skin. A study of 101 postmenopausal Japanese women taking either 10 mg or 30 mg daily of an isoflavone supplement or a placebo showed significant reduction in wrinkle area among those taking the supplement (at either dose) compared with the placebo group. There was also a significant difference in wrinkle depth between those taking the 30 mg supplement group and those taking the placebo.

In another study, healthy postmenopausal women taking either a drink containing isoflavone supplement or a placebo had detailed skin analyses after fifteen weeks. Those taking the supplements experienced a reduction in skin roughness and an average 10 percent greater decrease in wrinkle depth compared with the placebo group. The deeper the wrinkle initially, the greater the reduction, indicating that the supplements acted on the (deeper) dermal level of the skin. The results suggest that those with the deepest wrinkles may experience the greatest benefit. The analysis also showed an increase in collagen quantity and quality in the supplement group compared with the placebo group.

Flaxseed

Recent research suggests that consumption of flaxseed products can improve heart health, help prevent breast cancer, and even alleviate the annoying menopausal symptom of urinary incontinence.

One study showed that people with peripheral arterial disease consuming 30 grams of milled flaxseed every day for six months had significant reductions in blood pressure compared with those in a placebo group. These findings are supported by a recent review showing that flaxseed supplementation reduces blood pressure and that the effect may be greater when the whole seed is consumed on a long-term basis. Consumption of flaxseed may also help reduce cholesterol levels. A recent small study has shown that people consuming roasted flaxseed powder had an improved ratio of HDL ("good") to LDL ("bad") cholesterol after three months, compared with a group consuming a placebo.

Flaxseed also helps protect against breast cancer, according to the Ontario Women's Diet and Health Study, involving 2,999 women with breast cancer and a control group of 3,370 healthy women. Food questionnaires completed by both groups showed that weekly consumption of flaxseed or flax bread was associated with a reduction of approximately 20 percent in breast cancer risk.

Finally, results from the recent US National Health and Nutrition Examination Survey on consumption of flax lignans show that people who consumed higher levels of flax lignans (as measured by levels in the urine) had reduced levels of stress incontinence and other kinds of urinary incontinence. This benefit was not found with isoflavone phytoestrogen consumption.

Beating the Bloat

In addition to lost libido and vaginal dryness, women often suffer embarrassing digestive symptoms in menopause: bloating and gas. When our nutrient levels are depleted, our immune system, which protects us from toxins and disease agents, may be impaired. This can lead to the immune system's reacting to certain foods, like wheat, as toxic substances, and producing antibodies to them. These food sensitivities can cause or aggravate a variety of symptoms, including irritability, anxiety, constipation, abdominal bloating, diarrhea, excessive gas, irritable bowel syndrome, fatigue, depression, and insomnia. The good news is that these conditions can usually be reversed over a few months by increasing nutrient levels and removing problem foods from the diet, at least temporarily.

Quiz: Do You Suffer from Food Sensitivities?

- Do you suffer from constipation?
- Do you feel bloated after eating?
- Do you suffer from excessive gas?
- Do you suffer from diarrhea?
- Do you feel tired and depressed?
- Do you feel anxious for no apparent reason?
- Do you suffer from irritable bowel syndrome?

If you answered yes to more than two of these questions, you may have developed a temporary food sensitivity, likely to grains, in which case you should aim to cut them out of your diet for a while.

Transient food sensitivities may result in water retention, as the brain instructs the cells to retain fluid in an attempt to dilute the perceived toxic substances. The most common temporary sensitivity is to grains containing gluten, such as wheat, rye, barley, and oats (including the bran). Excluding these grains from the diet for a month or two can lead to rapid weight loss as the redundant fluid is eliminated from the body.

Typical Adverse Reactions to Gluten

- Diarrhea or constipation
- Excessive gas and abdominal bloating
- Headaches and irritability
- Weight gain
- Confusion
- Depression
- Mouth ulcers
- Skin rash
- Palpitations

Action Plan

Cut Them Out

Stop eating products containing wheat, oats, barley, and rye for four to six weeks. Most supermarkets and health food stores sell a wide range of wheat-free breads, crackers, pasta, pizza bases, muffins, cakes, and cookies (see the recommendations starting on page 170). See the list below for other grain- and gluten-containing foods to watch out for.

After four to six weeks, if your symptoms have improved, you can try reintroducing the various grains one by one. For example, choose one form of a particular grain, such as rye crackers. If you have no reaction after three days, choose another grain and repeat the process. Don't mix the grains, because if you get a reaction, you won't know which grain caused it. Keep careful notes to refer back to. It is best to reintroduce wheat last, as this grain is the most common source of problems.

Is It Forever?

Avoiding certain grains shouldn't be regarded as a life sentence. If you get a reaction to a grain, avoid eating it for a month or two before trying to reintroduce it. Wait until your body settles down, then try introducing another grain.

There is a distinction between food sensitivities and food allergies. Food sensitivities are often transient and easily corrected when nutrient levels are in an optimum range, whereas food allergies can be with us for life. Severe menopause symptoms are often caused by food sensitivities rather than allergies. A small number of women discover they have a permanent allergy to a particular food and soon realize they are better off avoiding that food altogether.

If your symptoms are severe, it is a good idea to give your body a complete rest from foods that provoke reactions for at least two or three months. It can take as long as six months, or even a year, for your body to get back to normal and learn to cope again with foods that you previously eliminated.

Foods Containing Grains

A huge number of the foods we commonly eat contain grains. Next time you're in the supermarket, have a closer look at some of the labels. You may be surprised! Keep in mind, too, that bran products all come from grains and may trigger sensitivities.

Wheat: The most obvious foods containing wheat include bread, crackers, cookies, cakes, pasta, cereals, pastries, and wheat and mixed-grain flours. Wheat is also often found in prepared sauces, soups, and processed foods such as sausages. Check food labels carefully, as wheat is sometimes listed using terms such as *modified starch, rusk,* and *cereal filler.* Soy sauce also contains wheat. Substitute wheat-free tamari, a slightly thicker and less salty version of soy sauce.

Oats: These are often found in mixed-grain breakfast cereals (watch out for oat flakes), cookies, crackers, and mixed-grain breads.

Rye: This is found in rye bread (which may also contain wheat) and flatbreads such as Ryvita.

Barley: This is often found in canned or powdered soups as well as barley drinks and beer.

Ending Food Cravings

Another way food can trouble us in menopause is through cravings for both sweet and savory foods. No matter how firmly we resolve to eat healthy, the cravings may send us scurrying out after dark to make the impulse purchases that contribute to our expanding waistlines.

Craving food is very common. In a survey my team and I conducted in the United Kingdom of one thousand women, 75 percent of respondents acknowledged feeling food and drink cravings, with 60 percent of those admitting a weakness for chocolate. But the problem in the United States may be even worse: according to a study published in the *Yale Journal of Biology and Medicine*, 90 percent of Americans experience food and drink cravings. These cravings can get worse around the time of menopause, leading us to pile on the pounds and subsequently finding it next to impossible to lose that extra weight.

> Only weeks after I began Maryon's program I noticed a huge difference. My energy began to return, and the migraines lessened. As I progressed, my concentration returned, the headaches went completely, and I had an incredible amount of energy.
>
> — Anne Germany

There is often a physiological basis for cravings. The brain and the nervous system require a constant supply of good nutrients to function normally, but our stressful lives mean that we don't always eat as healthily as we should. We skip meals or eat on the run. As a result, our blood sugar levels drop, and we start to crave a glucose fix to give us energy. So we grab a bar of chocolate or a cookie. This may give us a surge of energy, but it's hardly nutritious. What's more, this energy buzz is usually temporary, so before too long we're craving something sweet again, and the cycle continues, playing havoc with our waistlines and our health.

The trick is to know how to break the cycle. And, as with alcohol, drugs, smoking, and other habits, this involves a period of withdrawal.

Action Plan

To control cravings, you need to ensure that your nutrients are in an optimal range, particularly magnesium, chromium, and the B vitamins (see chapter 4). It's also important to eat some protein at each meal, which helps even out your blood sugar levels. Monitor what you eat, making sure you eat regular meals. Giving your diet an overhaul and making a few tweaks can help keep your blood sugar levels balanced so that you're not always longing for your next chocolate fix. As a result, any excess weight will drop off. Here are some goals to aim for:

- Consume nutritious, protein-rich food — little and often.
- Eat breakfast, lunch, and dinner every day, with wholesome mid-morning and mid-afternoon snacks.
- Eat fresh, home-cooked, nutritious foods whenever possible.
- Eat naturally sweet foods, like dried and fresh fruit, nuts, and seeds.
- Relax while you're eating, and enjoy your food.
- Plan your meals and snacks in advance (bearing in mind that you may need an additional five hundred calories per day during the week before your period).
- Always shop for food after you have eaten, not when you are hungry.
- Cut out caffeinated drinks, including tea, coffee, and soft drinks (even if they're labeled as decaffeinated). These can affect your insulin and blood sugar levels. Large amounts of sugar added to tea or coffee can also contribute to unstable blood glucose. As an alternative to black tea, try rooibos (or red bush) tea, which is caffeine-free; for coffee alternatives, try the coffee substitutes available in health food shops.
- Concentrate on a diet rich in chromium, magnesium, and vitamins B and C, including whole grains, chile, black pepper, chicken, and bell peppers.
- Keep alcohol to a minimum for now. Apart from being high in calories, excess alcohol can cause liver damage and lead to significant hypoglycemia (low blood sugar). Going out for drinks after work and then forgetting to eat dinner, for example, can cause a spike and subsequent fall in blood glucose levels, leading to headache, irritability, and other symptoms of hypoglycemia.

Quiz: Do Food and Drink Cravings Have a Hold over You?

- Are you embarrassed about the amount of chocolate and cookies you consume?
- Do you graze on chocolate, cookies, and chips throughout the day?
- Do you make impulse purchases of junk food?
- Do you take sugar in your tea or coffee?
- Do you drink more than three soft drinks per week (including diet drinks)?

- Do you routinely eat sweet food after your evening meal is complete?
- Have you been guilty of eating the children's chocolate or treats?
- Do you prefer chocolate to sex?
- Do you have a stash of comfort food?
- If you don't have chocolate at home, do you sometimes go out especially to buy some?
- Do you eat cookies, cake, fruit pies, desserts, or other food containing sugar most days?
- Do you eat more than three bars of chocolate a week?
- Have you ever bought chocolate as a gift, then eaten it yourself?
- Do you regularly consume ice cream?
- Do you crave salty foods like potato chips, salted nuts, or soy sauce?
- Do you feel hooked on certain types of food?
- Do you binge eat?
- Have you ever eaten chocolate and hidden the wrappers so that no one else knows?
- Do you use alcohol as a comfort?
- Do you find yourself consuming alcohol every day?

If you answered yes to three or more of these questions, you need to take action. Five yes responses mean things are out of your control, and more than six means you have some serious cravings to address! But there is a solution, so don't panic.

Nutrients for Beating Cravings

The key to beating food cravings is making sure you are getting enough of the nutrients that help keep your blood glucose at optimal levels. Magnesium is the most common deficiency among women, and B vitamins and chromium are also often in short supply.

Sufficient quantities of these important nutrients can be obtained from food, but you have to know where to look for them. You may also want to consider taking a specially formulated nutritional supplement that regulates blood sugar levels. For example, a Chromium Complex supplement, which contains B vitamins, vitamin C, and magnesium as well as chromium, is available through the web shop at maryonstewart.com.

Other nutrients that have been shown to reduce cravings include fish oils, which are thought to enhance insulin sensitivity. Extracts from the plant *Gymnema sylvestre*, a woody climbing shrub native to India and Africa, are thought to decrease the absorption of sugar through the intestine, but they are not suitable to take if you are diabetic or having surgery. Coenzyme Q10, a fat-soluble, vitamin-like substance that occurs naturally in the body, has been found to be critical for carbohydrate utilization and regulation of insulin at a dose of 60–200mg daily.

Lilly's Story

Lilly was a successful businesswoman who was struggling to function at work and at home when she first contacted me.

I felt I was falling apart at the time of my perimenopause, and I was unable to cope anymore. I lacked motivation. I was suffering with lack of sleep, mainly because of night sweats, and I had daytime hot flashes, anxiety, and brain fog. The emotional ups and downs left me feeling tearful, and migraines were costing me valuable workdays. I cut myself off from many friends, as I didn't feel up to being sociable. I started to feel very low about life, which just isn't who I am. I am normally a very positive, upbeat, bubbly person, and I began to think that person had gone.

I was plagued by migraines pretty much most months, which were taking several workdays a month. The night sweats were really bad, which then caused me huge amounts of insomnia, and I was struggling most days with a lack of sleep. My symptoms really affected my work because I run my own business, and I was finding it difficult to function on so little sleep, with the migraines and foggy brain, and just feeling really, really low, with high anxiety. It really got me down and I was struggling to keep running my company, and I couldn't share it with anyone who worked with me.

I actually saw two doctors, and to be honest I didn't get a lot of support. I was pretty much told that if I wanted HRT, I should go away and do my own research. Then if I decided I wanted it, I should go back and they would prescribe it.

I saw an advertisement on Facebook and signed up for Maryon's virtual class. It was *there that I heard about her six-week course, and I signed up immediately. Within a few weeks, I began to feel so much better. I was truly amazed. Within the six weeks of the course I had none of the symptoms and was sleeping through the night again.*

Since embarking on Maryon's program I feel like a completely different person. It's like someone pressed the reset button, and I'm once again the person I was! My husband completely agrees. I've got more clarity. I feel that I can be clear about what I want. I'm much happier. I'm more motivated, and I've now changed my career for a better life balance, and I feel so much happier about how my life is now.

Moving into week 4, we focus on science-based supplements that have been shown to be both safe and effective, how exercise is medicine, and how relaxation helps to curb hot flashes and night sweats.

Chapter 4

WEEK FOUR

Supplements, Exercise, and Relaxation

I know we would love a magic pill that would cure all the troubles of menopause, but the truth is it doesn't exist. There are so many things going on in the body at this time in our lives that managing symptoms requires a multipronged approach. Here I present a range of well-researched, safe, science-based dietary supplements that have been shown to relieve a wide variety of menopause symptoms. We know that exercise helps, too. If you're not already getting regular exercise, I show you how to get started on a program of gentle, enjoyable movement that can boost your health, improve your sleep, and lift your mood. Finally, I look at ways to make time for a dedicated period of relaxation each day. Used in combination, these approaches can help you go from feeling like a shadow of your former self to feeling better than you can remember.

Natural Dietary Supplements and Other Remedies

We've talked about the importance of including more nutrients in your diet when you hit perimenopause and menopause, but sometimes it just isn't possible to achieve the desired balance of nutrients through diet alone. However, you can easily make up for any shortfall with a selection of carefully chosen supplements.

By using supplements in addition to dietary changes, you can control hot flashes and night sweats much faster. Before I started recommending supplements that contained naturally occurring estrogen in my five-month program, it used to take at least three or four months to control hot flashes and night sweats. Once we included them, women began experiencing significant improvements within one month of their initial consultation.

It is vitally important to choose supplements that provide standardized amounts of active ingredients, as verified by independent testing. (Unfortunately the amount of active ingredients in many isoflavone-rich supplements, for example, varies considerably from that stated on the label.) The Six-Week Natural Menopause Solution recommends supplements that have undergone properly conducted clinical trials.

Research shows that supplements containing isoflavones and the herbs maca, St. John's wort, and black cohosh can be effective in controlling physical, cognitive, and emotional symptoms of menopause. They even get a special mention in the Health Economics Appendix of the current National Institute for Health and Care Excellence, known as the NICE guidelines in the UK. In the US, the North American Menopause Society acknowledges that herbs like black cohosh, red clover, St. John's wort, and dong quai (*Angelica sinensis*) have a place in the treatment of menopause symptoms.

Depending on your symptoms, there are several supplements that may benefit you. Use the chart on page 82 to help decide which supplements to try. Some are new to the market and not widely available but can be purchased online at maryonstewart.com /shop. Others are also available at pharmacies and health food stores.

When and How to Take Your Supplements

Always introduce supplements gradually. For example, if the recommended dosage is two to four capsules per day, start by taking one capsule a day and gradually build up to the recommended dose over a week or two. Supplements should always be taken after meals, unless otherwise specified.

Most of the supplements recommended here are compatible with prescription medications. In fact, after you start taking them, you may feel you have less need for medication. But don't change the dose of any prescribed drug without consulting your doctor, and always check with your doctor before taking St. John's wort or other herbs, as they may interact with medications such as antidepressants.

What about the Long Term?

How long you continue to take supplements is up to you. Once you have specific menopause symptoms under control, you may choose to gradually reduce the amount you are taking. If the symptoms return, you can always increase the dosage again.

Some supplements provide benefits over the long term, such as those that protect bone health. The risk of loss of bone mass is highest during the first five years after menopause, but it remains significant in the following ten years. If you are at risk of osteoporosis, you may need to continue to take supplements and also have a bone density scan every few years. For more on boosting bone density, see chapter 10.

Whether you should continue to take isoflavone-rich supplements depends on the amount of isoflavones you include in your diet. If you enjoy eating soy products, you will likely settle into a routine that will reduce your need for these supplements in the long term. It is advisable to continue with an isoflavone-rich regimen for the rest of your days to protect your bones, heart, and cognitive function.

Multivitamin and Mineral Supplements

To alleviate your most severe symptoms, the best option is to take a multivitamin and mineral supplement that contains good amounts of the essential nutrients mentioned in previous chapters. I recommend Gynovite Plus, which was formulated by Guy Abraham, a professor of obstetrics and gynecology in the US, especially for women from menopause onward. Clinical trials have found that it helps get nutrient levels back into an optimum range, improving hormone balance and bone density. The equivalent product in the UK is Fema 45+. Here I discuss other supplements that you might consider, in order of their relevance to common menopausal symptoms.

Some of the products I recommend are not widely available in stores but can be ordered from my online shop at maryonstewart.com/shop.

Isoflavone-Rich Supplements

If your symptoms are severe, a combination of a phytoestrogen-rich diet and isoflavone-rich supplements is likely to bring good results in the shortest time. For many years I have recommended the isoflavone-rich supplement Promensil, which is a standardized product containing extract of red clover. It contains high concentrations of the isoflavones genistein, daidzein, formononetin, and biochanin. Red clover is the richest known source of these four isoflavones, with up to ten times more of these isoflavones than the next richest source, soy. Promensil is designed to deliver the same daily dose of isoflavones as a vegetarian diet based on legumes (the tablets, which come in two strengths, contain approximately 40 or 80 mg total of the four isoflavones). Taking red clover in pill form is the only way you are likely to get an adequate amount, especially if you don't digest soy products very well.

There are many soy-based isoflavone supplements on the market, but they vary in quality. Phyto Soya capsules, produced by Arkopharma, are standardized and contain 35 mg of isoflavones per capsule. An international study published in *Menopause Journal* in 2007 showed that after one year of consumption, this product had no thickening effect on the lining of the uterus (a change that may be associated with cancer). Other studies have found similar conclusions with respect to breast tissue.

Another interesting group of products that turned up during my latest literature search is produced under the brand name Estromineral. Estromineral and Estromineral Serena are dietary supplements based on soy isoflavones and magnolia extract. In addition, they contain calcium, magnesium, and vitamin D3 to help maintain healthy bones, along with lactobacillus (a beneficial microbe also found in yogurt). These useful bacteria break down the soy isoflavones before they reach the small intestine, allowing the body to digest them better and absorb them more fully.

Femarelle, also known as DT56a, is a combination of soy, flax, vitamin B2 (riboflavin), and vitamin B7 (biotin). A few trials have shown encouraging results. In one study, over 80 percent of the participants taking Femarelle reported that the number of hot flashes they experienced diminished, and 38 percent reported a decrease in severity of the flashes. One study also found that the product had a similar effect on vaginal tissues to HRT, reducing dryness.

Hormone-Balancing Femmenessence

Another way of alleviating menopause symptoms is to help the hormone-producing glands in the body to function normally. I recommend a supplement called Femmenessence MacaPause, which has been shown in a number of studies to be a safe natural alternative to HRT. Femmenessence MacaPause is the first herbal product to be made from organic maca root, which has been grown for more than two thousand years in Peru. It has been shown in trials to raise levels of estrogen and progesterone, the two key hormones whose production falls at the time of perimenopause. Clinical trials have shown that it can bring about an 84 percent reduction in menopausal symptoms. Women report fewer hot flashes and night sweats, and improved sleep, energy levels, mood, and libido.

Femmenessence works by stimulating the hormone-secreting glands in the body, such as the pituitary and adrenal glands. By increasing the amount of estrogen and progesterone the body produces, it has a positive effect on bone health and cholesterol levels. There are two versions of Femmenessence. The perimenopausal product is called MacaLife, while the one for women who haven't had a period for a year is called MacaPause.

Fish Oils

Fish oils have been the subject of many clinical trials. They are derived from fish such as salmon, herring, sardines, anchovies, and mackerel. These are known as oily fish because they store significant quantities of oil in their tissues and belly fat; they are sometimes composed of up to 30 percent oil by weight. In addition to relieving joint pain, supplements derived from fish oils can help to raise mood, reduce the risk of heart disease, lower blood pressure, and maintain mental clarity. In a survey of over 1,200 women, my team and I discovered that women who consumed oily fish regularly had more energy and higher libido.

Fish oil contains both docosahexaenoic acid (DHA) and eicosapentaenoic acid (EPA). These omega-3 essential fatty acids (EFAs) have numerous roles in the body, from maintaining skin quality and regulating hormone function to preventing heart disease. They may even have a role in preventing dementia. If you are achy and lacking energy, libido, and mental clarity, you might consider taking a good-quality fish oil supplement as well as consuming oily fish. Efamol, the company that has led the way with research on EFAs over the years, has recently launched a new product called Efamol Active Memory, aimed at protecting and improving brain function. It contains high-strength omega-3 fish oils as well as folic acid, vitamin B12, ginkgo biloba, and phosphatidylserine, which is a fatty substance that protects the cells in our brain and helps to carry messages between them, possibly helping to preserve memory. The Efamol oils come from very sustainable fish stocks, and each batch is standardized.

Black Cohosh

The well-known herb black cohosh (*Actaea racemosa* or *Cimicifuga racemosa*) has been through several positive clinical trials, mostly with the Remifemin brand. It has been shown to reduce menopausal symptoms such as hot flashes and night sweats.

There has been debate about the effect of black cohosh on liver health. Although adverse effects have not been reliably documented, I tend not to recommend black cohosh as a first-line treatment, and it is not recommended for women who have had breast cancer.

However, if other treatments for menopausal symptoms are not effective, you might consider trying 20 mg of black cohosh twice a day for six months. It's especially useful for women who are sensitive to soy.

Vaginal Gels

In addition to dietary supplements, topical preparations can be useful for addressing vaginal dryness. Membrasin® Vaginal Vitality Cream, which is new to the US market, is registered in Europe as a medical device. It has been shown to be effective in hydrating as well as nurturing and maintaining vaginal tissues at the time of menopause and beyond. It is an all-natural product with a proprietary formula called SBA24®, a derivative of sea buckthorn.

Another phytoestrogen-rich herb, *Pueraria mirifica,* long used in Thailand for medicinal purposes, has also been shown to help with vaginal dryness. In a recent twelve-week study of eighty-two postmenopausal women suffering with vaginal dryness and atrophy, *Pueraria mirifica* vaginal gel was shown to significantly reduce symptoms. In another study in which it was compared with estrogen gel, it was shown to be equally effective in reducing symptoms over six months.

The company AH! YES makes a range of vaginal products derived from organic aloe and flaxseed that contain no synthetic products, hormones, or parabens. Both oil- and water-based vaginal gels are available. My clients generally prefer the water-based version for regular application. A newer product, AH! YES vaginal moisturizing gel is designed to match the typical vaginal environment, with none of the skin-damaging or concerning chemicals typically found in vaginal moisturizers. Many women find that it relieves vaginal dryness and alleviates irritation, itching, and burning.

Unlike the phytoestrogen gels, which sometimes have a recommended limit of twice-weekly application for long-term use, AH! YES products can be used as frequently as needed. I usually suggest clients use AH! YES on the days when they don't use the phytoestrogen gel, while their partner uses the oil-based product during intercourse while they are still healing their tissues.

Relief for Urinary Tract Infections

Urinary tract infections (UTIs) can be caused by bacterial infection, physical damage to the urogenital area, and nutritional deficiencies, including magnesium and vitamin D. It's thought that over half of all women get UTIs at some point, but they can occur more frequently at midlife, particularly after sexual intercourse. (See chapter 5 for advice on preventing UTIs.) Thinning tissues in the lining of the urethra at the time of menopause make some women much more vulnerable to recurrent infections.

As well as an adequate intake of magnesium and Vitamin D, I recommend the supplement D-mannose to women who experience UTIs. It is a plant-based substance found in cranberries, peaches, apples, and other fruits. Trials suggest that it may work by preventing bacteria from adhering to the lining of the urethra. Women who suffer regularly with UTIs can take it daily as a preventative measure. When an infection occurs, D-mannose can be taken regularly throughout the day until the discomfort has passed. I recommend the Solaray brand, which contains 400 mg of CranActin cranberry extract in addition to 1,000 mg of D-mannose. (If you suffer with recurrent UTIs or your symptoms are severe, consult your doctor, as prolonged UTIs can lead to kidney infection.)

Ristela / Lady Prelox

Called Ristela in the US and Lady Prelox in the UK, this dietary supplement containing pycnogenol pine bark extract, the amino acids L-arginine and L-citrulline, and Rosvita rose hip extract has been shown to help women feel sexy again at midlife. A study of premenopausal women suggested that supplementation with Lady Prelox improves sexual function and enjoyment. Two pilot studies have been conducted on women of menopausal age focusing on desire, arousal, lubrication, orgasm, satisfaction, and pain. The results were encouraging enough for larger studies to be recommended. None of the ingredients have hormone-like effects, and the individual components have been on the market for years.

Other Useful Herbs

A number of other herbs can help relieve symptoms of both perimenopause and menopause. Some are discussed in more depth in chapter 5. Many of these herbs are available at maryonstewart.com/shop.

> **Licorice root (*Glycyrrhiza glabra*):** Licorice root contains phytoestrogens and can be used in conjunction with other herbs and brewed into herbal tea. However, licorice can cause sodium retention and increases the risk of high blood pressure in some people and may also have a laxative effect.

Dong quai (*Angelica sinensis*): This herb contains phytoestrogens and is considered in Chinese medicine to be a harmonizing tonic. It has traditionally been used to treat female complaints, such as heavy menstrual bleeding and PMS, and now has a place in the treatment of menopause symptoms.

Sage leaf (*Salvia officinalis*): This member of the mint family contains estrogenic substances that can help relieve hot flashes and night sweats. In a study carried out on the medicinal uses of plant drugs, forty patients were given dried aqueous extract of fresh sage (440 mg) and forty were given infusion of sage (4.5 g) daily. Both groups of patients experienced a reduction in sweating.

Vitex (*Vitex agnus-castus*): Vitex, sometimes known as the chaste tree, is a flowering shrub that is native to the Mediterranean and Central Asia. Research shows it can significantly relieve symptoms of PMS and perimenopause, such as irritability, mood swings, headaches, breast fullness, abdominal cramps, and depression. Results are usually noticeable within three cycles.

Valerian (*Valeriana officinalis*): Valerian root is a traditional herbal remedy for symptomatic relief of stress and tension, promoting natural sleep without the sometimes unpleasant side effects of more conventional drugs. It can also be taken for anxiety and conditions worsened by stress, such as irritable bowel syndrome.

Ginseng (*Panax ginseng*): Ginseng root can be helpful in controlling hot flashes, especially when taken in conjunction with 400 IU of vitamin E. A dose of 500 mg of ginseng twice a day for four weeks has been shown to improve sexual function and quality of life as well as mitigating menopause symptoms.

St. John's wort (*Hypericum perforatum*): This herb, long used to treat depression, has fewer side effects than conventional antidepressants. It is thought to be effective in treating moderate rather than severe depression. In addition, a twelve-week German study of 111 women experiencing libido problems at the time of menopause found that 60 percent of the women using St. John's wort regained their libido significantly.

Note: Although St. John's wort is an effective supplement, it is not compatible with antidepressants. I never advise women to begin taking it until they have weaned themselves off antidepressants in consultation with their doctor.

Danielle's Story

Danielle was a senior manager who was struggling to function because of her menopause symptoms. She was due to get married and was afraid of what the future had in store.

I couldn't function on a daily basis at all. I was in a lot of pain. My joints were aching. I wasn't sleeping. I had lots of brain fog, which was very scary, and I just couldn't function at work. I had a very responsible job and had to go in to work pretending, because I felt like I was wading through mud. In the afternoons especially, all I wanted was to crash. I'd love to have just gone to bed and slept for the afternoon. My hot flashes were awful. I felt very anxious, which was made worse by the need to run out of meetings because I was bleeding so heavily. It was just horrendous. I was given antidepressants by my doctor, but I wasn't depressed. He said they would work for the other symptoms, but they didn't, I just felt worse.

I was due to get remarried and knew that if my marriage was to be successful, I needed to get myself back into good shape. My fiancé bought me a ticket to Maryon Stewart's program, and I have never looked back.

I worked diligently to follow Maryon's advice during the six-week course and religiously took the supplements she recommended. Amazingly, I began to feel better quite quickly and noticed that I was losing weight without even dieting.

Now I'm able to function again. And, fortunately that happened right before my wedding, so I was able to enjoy the day and have a wonderful honeymoon. Honestly and truly, after a couple of weeks of coming off the things I was not supposed to be eating, I started to see a change. After six weeks I was sleeping better, and my headaches had gone. I used to suffer from migraines every month, but I haven't had one now for ages. My brain fog has lifted, which is so important for me, as I feel I can function again, and I feel excited about being able to remember things again. My joint aches have improved, I can sleep peacefully — which is huge — and I feel lighter.

I feel better than I can remember. I get up in the mornings with energy and enthusiasm. I'm usually up by 6:30 a.m., and I'm active instead of wanting desperately to stay in bed for the day. I'm doing things I thought I would never do again, and I'm painting as well as working and loving my work life. Before Maryon's program it was all about the burden of my symptoms, and now it's all about my life: living it joyfully.

Choosing Supplements

The table below summarizes recommendations and dosages of supplements for many menopausal symptoms. When taking supplements, it's important to follow the instructions on the label unless you are getting expert advice.

Problem	Recommended Supplement(s)	Daily Dose
General symptoms of menopause	In US: Gynovite Plus multivitamin and mineral supplement In UK: Fema 45+	2–4 tablets per day 2 tablets per day
Hot flashes and night sweats	Isoflavone-rich supplements, such as Promensil, Phyto Soya, or Femmenessence MacaPause	1–2 tablets per day (40–80 mg of isoflavones)
	In US: Remifemin Black Cohosh In UK: Niteherb	2 tablets per day 1 tablet per day
	Sage leaf	300–900 mg per day
Vaginal dryness	In US: Membrasin® SBA24® In UK: Omega 7 SBA24	2 capsules once per day
	Remifemin FeuchtCreme (see chapter 5)	Nightly for the first 30 nights, then as needed
Low libido and depression	St. John's wort	900 mg per day (dosage depends on capsule size)
Aches and pains	Glucosamine and chondroitin or joint-health supplements that contain MSM (methylsulfonylmethane), rosehip, and ginger	1,100–2,000 mg glucosamine per day and 300–200 mg chondroitin per day (follow dosage directions on label)
	Fish oils	750 mg twice daily
	Vitamin D	1,000–4,000 IU daily

Problem	Recommended Supplement(s)	Daily Dose
Loss of libido	Horny goat weed (see chapter 5)	600 mg per day
	Femmenessence MacaPause	2 capsules twice daily, morning and night
	In US: Ristela In UK: Lady Prelox	2 tablets a day with meals
Osteoporosis	Promensil, Femmenessence MacaPause, and AlgaeCal or Osteoguard (see chapter 10)	Follow label directions
Urinary tract infection	Solaray D-mannose	1 tablet per day (or more as needed)
Insomnia	Valerian	600 mg at night
Controlling heavy periods and associated anemia	Magnesium citrate	2 × 150 mg tablets daily
	Vitex agnus-castus	1,000 mg
	Iron (as ferrous sulfate)	1 × 200 mg tablet with fruit juice

The Value of Exercise

The benefits of exercise for menopausal symptoms cannot be overstated. Increased mental alertness, more energy and vitality, the ability to perform daily tasks without getting breathless or tired, greater flexibility, faster reaction times, increased immunity and stronger bones are just some of them. Exercise is also a great stress buster. Achieving these benefits requires time and effort, but this is a small price to pay for such huge rewards.

It's even more important to be positive about exercise now than when you were younger. Anything that gets you moving will help improve your energy levels and reduce symptoms of depression, anxiety, and insomnia, as well as boost your confidence, self-esteem, and well-being.

Aerobic exercise — anything that increases your heart rate and breathing rate — helps protect against heart disease. Weight-bearing exercise — moderate-impact activities

After taking supplements and including naturally occurring estrogen regularly in my diet, I began to feel so much better. By the end of the six weeks the severe night sweats were almost gone and I was sleeping much better. Heaven!

— Andrea Bauer

in which you support your own body weight, such as walking, jogging, dancing, or tennis, and working your upper body through strength training — helps strengthen your bones and protects against osteoporosis. Simply dancing to your favorite music will help release endorphins (the feel-good hormones) and speed up your metabolism, helping shed the extra pounds we tend to gain at midlife. (See page 88 for specific exercise recommendations.)

Exercise is particularly important at the time of menopause, as our metabolism (the rate at which the body burns calories) tends to slow down as we get older. When you were young, you could probably eat what you liked without gaining much weight, but now you may only have to look at a doughnut to pile on the pounds, especially around the middle.

Exercise helps in several ways. First, you burn more calories while you're doing it, and it can also increase your metabolic rate for up to twenty-four hours afterwards. Second, regular exercise, particularly strength or resistance training (which includes activities like Pilates, yoga, swimming, and cycling, as well as weight training), builds muscle. The greater your muscle mass, the higher your metabolic rate, and the more calories you burn even when you're not exercising.

Making exercise part of our everyday lifestyle helps to protect us from heart disease and dementia as well as building new bone. Not exercising makes us feel old before our time.

Exercise Decreases

- LDLs, the "bad" cholesterol
- Heart disease risk
- Blood pressure
- Body fat
- Anxiety, stress, and depression
- Type 2 diabetes risk

Exercise Increases

- HDLs, the "good" cholesterol
- Oxygen transport
- Aerobic capacity
- Circulation
- Bone mass and density
- Reaction speed
- Coordination
- Energy levels
- Overall well-being

If you haven't enjoyed exercising in the past, you're probably already groaning, but I promise you will reap enormous benefits from getting up and moving. Many women who started exercise for the first time as part of my program have come to absolutely love it. Exercise also improves your circulation, so your skin will look better, and you'll feel radiant.

Don't worry, you're not expected to run a marathon (unless you want to, of course). You're not competing with anyone but yourself. The aim is to improve your level of fitness gradually over several months.

Quiz: How Fit Are You?

- Do you exercise more than three times a week for more than thirty minutes at a time?
- Does it take a lot of exercise before you feel out of breath?
- Can you run up and down a flight of stairs without panting?

If you answered no to more than two of these questions, it's time to get moving! Remember to enter your score on your Natural Menopause Solution worksheet.

Cautions

- Check with your doctor before starting any exercise program if you haven't exercised for a long time, or if you suffer from heart disease, have high blood pressure, have joint or back problems, are very overweight, have a serious illness, or are convalescing.

- Before performing any exercises in your home or garden, check that the location is safe and that the surfaces are not wet or slippery.
- Ensure that any supports and equipment you use are strong enough to take your weight.
- Make sure you start out warm enough. Layered, loose clothing that you can remove easily as you heat up is ideal.
- Wait at least an hour after meals before exercising, and drink plenty of water to avoid dehydration.

Action Plan

Choosing Activities

The first rule of exercise is to choose activities you enjoy. If you already like walking, this is a great way to start. If you can't think of any form of exercise that appeals to you, think back to activities you enjoyed when you were younger. Maybe you were a keen tennis player, swimmer, dancer, or roller skater. There are more and more activities on offer today for people of all ages, so you should be able to find something that suits you.

You may prefer to exercise with other people. This might mean joining an exercise or dance class or going for a jog with a friend. If you prefer (or are required) to stay at home, select a good home exercise session on YouTube, or simply dance or sing to your favorite music. Whatever it takes and whatever you fancy, you have already jumped the most difficult hurdle — you've taken the first step in creating an exercise program.

Once you start, it's a good idea to vary the type of exercise you do on different days of the week to target different parts of your body and help stave off boredom. Good options include running, power walking, cycling, swimming, using the cardio machines at the gym, tennis, Zumba, Pilates, dancing, jumping rope, and aerobics.

Alternatively, you can just stretch and dance to your favorite music. I tune in to a rock station and do a workout before the day begins, and I swear I feel twenty years younger as a result. If you haven't got an established exercise routine, why not give it a try?

You can also incorporate exercise into your daily life. Use the stairs instead of the elevator. Walk or ride a bike instead of driving or using public transport. Use a Hula Hoop in the evening instead of sitting watching TV. Walk around while you are talking to friends on the phone. If you do your own housework, put real effort into it while playing your favorite music.

How Long and How Often?

The second rule of exercise is to start slowly to avoid discomfort or injury, especially if you're not used to exercise. "Little and often" should be the rule. The adage "No pain, no gain" is outdated. Exercise does not have to be hell to be healthy. You should feel invigorated at the end of your activity, but not exhausted. Listen to your body. Sometimes you will have plenty of energy and feel you can tackle anything, and sometimes you won't. The secret is not to push yourself too hard — just do as much as you feel comfortable with.

If you haven't been a regular exerciser for a while, it's going to take time to rebuild your stamina. Take one day at a time and try to gradually increase the time and intensity of your exercise sessions each week. If you feel stressed, or have high levels of cortisol (the stress hormone), begin with gentle exercise, as vigorous aerobic exercise can make you feel worse.

Keep the benefits of exercise uppermost in your mind until you have established a regular routine. When you reach your goal of four or five exercise sessions a week, try to stick to it. There's no need to do more — too much exercise can strain your joints and bones.

After each workout, tap into how you are feeling. Exercise encourages your body to release endorphins, the body's own feel-good hormones, which can make you feel elated, full of energy, and proud of yourself. Hold on to that feeling, and next time you start talking yourself out of exercising, remind yourself how good it makes you feel.

Taking Care of Your Body while Exercising

- Warm up slowly for the first few minutes.
- Don't push yourself too hard. It's not a competition: you're just trying to increase your own fitness over time. If you're struggling or have concerns about increasing your level of exercise, check with your doctor or fitness trainer.
- Cool down gradually, rather than stopping suddenly.

Within twelve weeks of starting an exercise regimen, you will feel more energetic, be able to cope more effectively with stress, sleep better, fight off infections more successfully, and generally feel a whole lot better.

The Challenges of Exercise

If you're not used to exercise, you may experience some surprises. First, if you start to sweat, it's not just another hot flash, but a sign that your body is using up energy and needs to get rid of the excess heat it is producing. Sweating does not mean you're unfit: it means you're getting fit! And the fitter you become, the less you'll sweat.

You may huff and puff as you begin to exercise. As long as you can still carry on a conversation and are not struggling to breathe, this should be nothing to worry about. It just means you're working! Take it at your own pace: it's not a race, just a process of improving your fitness over time.

Simple Exercise Options

Warm-Up Moves

Whatever type of exercise you choose, warm up before you start. This helps get you in the mood and also increases blood flow to your muscles, providing more oxygen to fuel your activities. Walking, gentle jogging, marching on the spot, stationary cycling, or any activity that uses your large muscle groups is good for warming up.

Move your joints through their full range of movement to loosen them up and gently stretch the muscles you are about to use. Try to hold your stretches for six to eight seconds, and avoid bouncing, which can strain cold muscles.

Cool-Down Moves

Exercise increases your heart rate, making you breathe faster and more deeply, which is good for heart health. But in the same way as you use gears to gradually slow down a car, it is much better to come out of exercise gradually, rather than stopping suddenly. Cool off by slowing your pace and walking around after exercising.

Gently stretch the muscles that you have been using, to keep them flexible. Try to build in some relaxation time at the end of your session to reward yourself for your efforts and to give you time to release tension.

Pelvic Floor Exercises

One set of muscles that needs special attention is the pelvic floor muscles. These get weaker with pregnancies and as we age. We need to keep them toned to prevent urinary incontinence. Women with low levels of vitamin D are more likely to have pelvic floor disorders and urinary incontinence, so if you experience these problems it might be an idea to ask your doctor to measure your levels.

You could benefit from pelvic floor exercise at menopause, especially if:

- You suffer with stress incontinence, meaning that every time you laugh, cough, or sneeze you leak a few drops of urine.
- You have difficulty getting to the bathroom in time and notice that you are leaking when going about ordinary life.

See Working Your Pelvic Floor Muscles on page 26 for an effective way to strengthen these muscles. You can do these exercises anywhere. I sometimes do mine while driving my car!

If you struggle to work your pelvic floor, there are useful gadgets that can help you to strengthen your muscles, like Elvie and Kegel Fit, which come with apps to monitor your progress. Pilates, with its focus on working the body's core muscles, also develops pelvic floor strength.

What the Research Says

A new Finnish study shows that women in menopause who were physically active had less depression and anxiety, fewer hot flashes and night sweats, and a greater sense of well-being than those who were less active. This finding is backed up by a report from Latin America showing the dangers of a sedentary lifestyle in menopause, including heart disease, obesity, and osteoporosis.

A recent study from the University of Kansas Medical Center suggests that moderate aerobic exercise also improves cognitive function. Another study shows that small amounts of exercise — even below the recommended levels — increase the lifespan of people over the age of sixty. A study involving aerobic exercise showed that it helps relieve sleep problems during menopause.

In another study, women who undertook a twelve-week walking and jogging program felt better, enjoyed social functions more, participated in more activities, and were less tired at the end of the day than a control group.

Exercise has been shown to reduce symptoms of depression and anxiety more effectively than psychotherapy. In a comparative study, after twelve weeks, women who participated in aerobics had fewer symptoms of depression and anxiety than women who had psychotherapy. At a follow-up session one year later, this was still the case.

Exercise may even slow the aging of the central nervous system. People who exercise regularly are consistently more alert and have faster reaction times. It has also been shown that the fitter people are, the more mental clarity they have.

According to a study published in the *Journal of Advanced Nursing*, regular exercise can reduce severe menopausal symptoms and improve quality of life. Researchers from the University of Granada in Spain found that the number of women suffering severe symptoms dropped nearly 25 percent after they began a twelve-month supervised exercise program consisting of cardiovascular, stretching, strengthening, and relaxation exercises, while symptoms worsened among women who didn't exercise.

A survey of the physical activity level of a group of 305 women aged between forty-five and sixty, at various stage of menopause, reveals that higher levels of physical activity were associated with reduced likelihood of severe urogenital symptoms. The researchers found that 11 percent of women with low physical activity levels reported symptoms, compared with 4 percent of those with high physical activity levels. Sustained, regular aerobic exercise, such as swimming, walking, cycling, and running, tends to be most effective for relieving symptoms.

Relaxation Techniques

The flip side of exercise is rest and relaxation, which also have huge benefits at this time of life, especially for women with busy or stressful lives. And luckily the ability to be still, experience gratitude, and appreciate beauty in our surroundings is Mother Nature's gift to us. We can all do it, and it costs nothing, but it pays huge dividends. A daily twenty-minute relaxation session can reduce hot flashes by up to 60 percent.

When we are feeling stressed and wound up, relaxation may not come easily, or we may feel that we don't have time for it. But relaxation rests our brain, making it more efficient, as well as giving us an energy boost. As a bonus, it can reduce hot flashes by more than 50 percent.

It's not uncommon to find it difficult to switch off. In my experience formal relaxation or meditation quiets the mind, but it is an acquired skill. So don't be too hard on yourself if your mind keeps running in the fast lane when you first attempt to practice formal relaxation techniques. It's like building new muscles: it takes time.

You can choose from a whole range of practices and techniques to help you rest and relax. These include yoga, creative visualization, mindfulness meditation, qi gong, cognitive behavior therapy, and tai chi. In addition, there are apps, like *Pzizz* and *Headspace*, that can coach you through structured relaxation or meditation sessions or just provide a soothing audio background for relaxation.

Yoga

Yoga has been practiced for thousands of years. It works on the principle that mind and body need to be working in perfect harmony for optimal health. To help you achieve this, yoga uses asana (poses that relax muscles) and pranayama (breathing techniques that improve oxygen flow and calm the body). It is best to attend a yoga class to learn the basic poses and get feedback from an instructor; you can then practice at home on a regular basis.

Pilates

Pilates, developed in the 1920s, is another form of mind-body training. Pilates combines breathing techniques and exercises to develop strength, balance, coordination, bodily and spatial awareness, and flexibility. As with yoga, you should go to some classes to learn the technique before practicing at home.

Tai Chi

Tai chi, an ancient Chinese form of movement, was originally developed as a self-defense discipline but has evolved into a graceful form of exercise that can reduce stress and increase both physical and mental well-being. Often described as moving meditation, it involves a series of flowing movements performed in a slow and focused way, accompanied by deep breathing. It's a self-paced and gentle form of physical exercise.

Tai chi can improve posture, balance, flexibility, and strength. In addition, it has been shown to boost mood, reduce joint pain, strengthen the immune system, and improve heart health.

Mindfulness

In recent years mindfulness has become a popular practice. The founder of mindfulness meditation, Jon Kabat-Zinn, gives this definition: "Mindfulness means paying attention in a particular way: on purpose, in the present moment, and non-judgmentally." It can be practiced as we go about our day as well as during focused mindfulness meditation sessions.

Like many other disciplines, mindfulness is an acquired skill. There are many good mindfulness books and apps, including the Mindfulness Daily app, which cues you to pause at intervals during the day to practice mindfulness. Many research studies have shown that mindfulness has significant health benefits, including lowering levels of the stress hormone cortisol, reducing the prevalence of heart disease and depression, and even helping us at the time of menopause by reducing hot flashes and levels of anxiety and inducing more peaceful sleep.

Cognitive Behavior Therapy (CBT)

Cognitive behavioral therapy, or CBT, is a form of talking therapy and behavior modification based on the fact that thoughts, feelings, attitudes, actions, and physical well-being are all connected. If we change one of these, we can alter the others. It connects what we think to what we do.

When we feel worried or distressed, which are common feelings during menopause, we often fall into patterns of thinking and responding that can worsen how we feel. CBT can help us notice and change problematic thinking styles and behavior patterns. It is recommended by the North American Menopause Society as a low-risk treatment for hot flashes as well as other physical and psychological menopause symptoms.

Creative Visualization

This simple, enjoyable way to relax requires little or no training and is ideal if you are short on time. This is all you need to do:

1. Lie flat on the floor with your head supported — or, if you are at work or traveling, find a quiet space where you can sit and relax.
2. Bend your knees, keeping your feet flat on the floor.
3. Close your eyes, breathe steadily and slowly, while consciously relaxing your face, fingers, arms, legs, and toes.

4. Continue to breathe slowly and steadily. Start to visualize something you fancy — anything from a world cruise to a wonderful night out. The trick is to keep your mind focused on your fantasy for as long as you can. After fifteen to twenty minutes, bring yourself gently back to reality, rolling onto your side before standing up.

Creative visualization requires practice, and you may have to work at it before you feel the full benefits. If your mind is very busy, it can help to jot down your intrusive thoughts on paper before you start, so you can stay focused on your fantasy.

 ## LEARN TO LET GO

Try this simple exercise to release muscle tension. It only takes fifteen to twenty minutes.

Wear loose, comfortable clothes and find a warm, quiet place where you won't be interrupted. Put on some calming music to help you relax, and adjust the lighting so you feel comfortable. Lie down on the floor or your bed. Instead of focusing on the outside world and its problems, tune in to your body and become aware of your tension.

1. Place a pillow under your head and relax your arms and lower jaw.
2. Take a few slow, deep breaths.
3. Concentrate on tensing and relaxing the muscles in each part of your body, starting with the toes on one foot, then on the other foot. Gradually work your way up each leg, tensing and relaxing each ankle, then each calf and shin, each thigh, your gluteal and abdominal muscles, and so on up to your head (including arms and hands). Breathe deeply as you focus on each body part.
4. When you reach your head and your face feels relaxed, remain in this position for fifteen minutes.
5. Gradually allow yourself to return to awareness of your surroundings. Roll onto your side, sit up slowly, and sip a glass of water.

What the Research Says

Tai chi and yoga have a long record of improving health. A study at Tufts University showed that tai chi is as effective as physical therapy in relieving the pain caused by knee osteoarthritis. A recent review of clinical trials shows that both tai chi and qi gong have beneficial effects on the heart, quality of life, and bone health.

Yoga has been shown to help relieve menopausal symptoms. Research has shown that women who practice yoga are more likely to eat healthily as well.

A lesser-known practice called "laughter yoga" is being promoted by the US Administration on Aging, and a recent trial has shown very promising results. That's not a joke!

Research on CBT has also shown some benefits for women in menopause. CBT-Meno is a program consisting of education and cognitive and behavioral strategies for vasomotor and depressive symptoms, anxiety, sleep difficulty, and sexual concerns. A Canadian study of its effectiveness compared women undergoing therapy and a control group. After twelve weeks, the CBT-Meno group showed significantly greater improvements for all symptoms except anxiety compared with the control group. These findings suggest that CBT-Meno is effective in treating some menopausal symptoms.

> Menopause is an excellent time to take stock of the rest of your life, because at menopause you may only be halfway there.
>
> — Susan Wysocki,
> past president of the North American Menopause Society

Additionally, Iranian researchers reviewed the literature on the impact of CBT on menopausal symptoms. They divided the CBT approaches into direct face-to-face (individual and group) therapy and indirect (self-help) therapy. Symptoms were categorized as vasomotor, psychological, and organic disorders. Generally face-to-face CBT was more effective than self-help, and group CBT was more effective in treating psychological symptoms.

Finally, there is a lot of interest in mindfulness as an overall approach to improving both mental and physical health. Two recent studies show that mindfulness and related cognitive therapies can help with depression and hot flashes. Another report suggests that mindfulness is particularly helpful in addressing insomnia.

Next, in chapter 5, we'll focus on getting comfortable sex back on the menu, busting stress, and sleeping peacefully.

Chapter 5

WEEK FIVE

Sex, Stress, and Sleep

Putting Sex Back on the Menu

Your partner is still keen, but during menopause sex may be the last thing on your mind. You are not alone. Many women find that their desire for sex wanes as they approach menopause. Studies show that up to 75 percent of women feel their sex drive has declined since menopause. That's not surprising when up to 70 percent report suffering from vaginal dryness. Spontaneity and enjoyment understandably go out the window when penetration is painful.

Many women regard their loss of libido as part of their fading youth. Our libido levels are often a well-kept secret, and not something we consider an acceptable part of social chitchat over cocktails, even with our best friends. There are no standards for a normal level of libido, and there is no such thing as a normal sex drive. What is normal for one couple may be abnormal for another. You can judge your libido only by your own standards. If you are concerned that your sexual desire has diminished, the good news is you can take action to restore it.

Tiredness, lack of energy, and mood swings can put a strain on the most solid relationship. At the same time, falling levels of estrogen can result in the lining of your vagina becoming dry and uncomfortable. When this happens, penetration can become painful and, in extreme cases, the tissue may tear and bleed. If you are also suffering from night sweats, it's not surprising that you don't feel very sexy.

Many women suffer in silence, thinking this is an inevitable part of growing older. But it doesn't have to be this way. There are plenty of things you can do naturally to repair the vaginal lining, encourage the cells to produce mucus again, and rekindle your libido.

Quiz: How's Your Libido?

- Have you lost your sex drive?
- Do you have sex less often than you used to?
- Do you find sex painful?
- Does your vagina feel dry?
- Have you stopped looking forward to having sex?
- Have you stopped communicating with your partner on an intimate level?
- Are you too tired for sex?
- Has your enjoyment of sex diminished?
- Do you make excuses to avoid sex?

If you answered yes to more than two of these questions, try the following action plan to give your sex life a boost.

Causes of Loss of Libido

Low libido may have multiple causes, not all of which are related to menopausal changes. Excessive weight gain or weight loss, irregular periods, hair loss, or excessive hair growth may all signify hormonal problems that can result in a low sex drive. Other hormone disturbances, like thyroid problems or galactorrhea, a white milky discharge from the nipples, can also cause low libido, as can the hormonal changes at the time of menopause that cause night sweats and insomnia. Childbirth — now more common than it used to be among women approaching the age of menopause — also affects libido with rapid changes in hormone levels and disturbed sleep.

Sometimes women are put off sex because intercourse is too painful. The pain may be due to infection, vaginismus (spasm of the vaginal muscles), an enlarged or displaced uterus, or another hormonal abnormality. Additional causes of low libido include a history of long-term illness, lack of energy, and psychologically distressing past experiences.

Sex can also be offputting if it leads to urinary tract infections (UTIs). When the vaginal tissues are fragile, they can be damaged by pressure from penetration. This can make the urethra vulnerable to infection, especially if you are short of vitamin D and magnesium, two common deficiencies.

Stress, worry in the here and now, and depression often take their toll on sex drive. When you are mentally preoccupied with pressing problems, the body naturally diverts its energy to helping you through the troubled times, and sexual desire may take a back seat.

Herbal Helpers

The good news is that there is no need to accept falling libido levels as an inevitable part of aging. Energy levels often begin to wane prior to menopause, as estrogen levels decline and symptoms of estrogen withdrawal and long-term nutritional deficiencies start to show. Symptoms subside, and libido can be rekindled, once nutrient levels have been replenished and the body is supplied with naturally occurring phytoestrogens (see chapter 3). In addition, a number of traditional medicinal herbs contain active ingredients that can improve mood and raise energy levels and libido.

Maca root, cultivated in Peru, has been used as a safe aid to health for more than two thousand years. It stimulates the hormone-producing glands in the body. A few studies suggest that maca can alleviate sexual dysfunction, reduce vaginal dryness, and improve libido. There are thirteen different types of maca. Each has a different color and active ingredient content. Although most of them apparently work better for men than for women, maca has been shown to help to control menopause symptoms like hot flashes, night sweats, and fluctuating moods. It may also strengthen bones and improve sleep.

Ginseng is considered to be nonaddictive and far safer to use than stimulants, and is used to reduce the effects of stress, improve sexual performance, boost energy levels, enhance memory, and stimulate the immune system. It contains vitamins A and B6 and zinc, which helps the production of thymic hormones, necessary for the functioning of the immune system.

Ginseng is an adaptogen, which means that it has the ability to normalize body functions. For example, it helps to regulate blood sugar levels, which is of particular use in treating diabetes, and lowers blood pressure if it is too high.

St. John's wort has also been shown to help boost a waning libido. A German study published a few years ago, on a group of 111 women with libido problems before menopause, showed that 60 percent of the participants had regained their libido significantly after a twelve-week course of 900 mg of St. John's wort per day.

Horny goat weed (*Epimedium*, also known as barrenwort) has been used in traditional Chinese medicine for centuries. It has been shown to increase sexual interest in both men and women. Another herb, tribulus, thought to increase the production of testosterone in men and increase their sex drive, has also been shown to significantly boost libido in women.

Below the Belt: Vaginal Dryness

We've already talked a lot about dealing with hot flashes and night sweats. Many of the natural remedies recommended for those symptoms will reach our important little places too. But they do deserve a special mention, as vaginal and bladder symptoms at midlife and beyond can be devastating. When the vagina becomes a no-go area and our muscles and tissues let us down to the point of incontinence, it's not surprising that we are not going to love ourselves or feel sexy.

Just as the skin lines and protects the outside of the body, mucous membranes line and protect the respiratory and urogenital tracts and the inner surface of the eyes. They are important channels for interactions between the body and the environment; they are also the major routes by which pathogens, toxins, and allergens can enter the body. Thus, mucous membranes play an important role in health and the general well-being of the whole body. Mucous membranes, including the vaginal lining, are often damaged by diseases, stress, aging, and side effects of medications.

Understanding the causes of vaginal dryness is important. When we had plenty of circulating estrogen prior to perimenopause, most of us took vaginal lubrication for granted. The presence of estrogen in our fertile years ensures that there are plenty of new cells producing lubrication and maintaining the elasticity of the vaginal lining. However, when our estrogen levels fall at midlife, production at the cell factory diminishes, and our tissues dry out. The dryness can cause pain, as the thinning, brittle tissues can tear easily; some women even experience burning sensations and bleeding. But we can effectively turn the factory lights back on and get the production line up and running.

Paradoxical as it sounds, having regular intercourse can help. So can pelvic floor (Kegel) exercises (see page 26). Here's a guide to other solutions for vaginal dryness.

Diet

The first approach is dietary changes. We have already seen how we can replace our body's own supply of estrogen with phytoestrogens from food and supplements. Consuming

100 mg of isoflavones per day, little and often, will help fool the brain into thinking that there is once again plenty of circulating estrogen and restoring lubrication and elasticity to the vaginal tissues. Most of my clients notice a huge change within four to five months; some begin to notice improvements even before the end of the six-week course.

In addition to consuming isoflavones, you should make sure that your diet is healthy and balanced. Many women try to avoid fats altogether, but eating healthy fats is important. When you eat a healthy diet, your body is better equipped to make estrogen. Eliminating sugars and any foods that cause allergies is also important.

A few great dietary supplements can also alleviate vaginal dryness, such as the all-natural supplement Membrasin®, or Omega 7 SBA24 in the UK.

> Even after a month on Maryon's program, my dry vagina is wet again, and both my husband and I are delighted that sex is back on the menu. The hot flashes and night sweats are already greatly reduced, and unbelievably 80 percent of the joint pain that I have lived with practically my whole life has gone!
>
> — Lisa Finn

Hydration

Drinking plenty of water is extremely important for alleviating feminine dryness. Drinking at least eight glasses of water each day helps to keep the body from getting dehydrated, which can lead to more problems with vaginal dryness. And it costs almost nothing.

While you may think this is a pretty obvious idea, many women don't really think about it. If you are very dehydrated, lubrication is going to become a problem for your body. Alcoholic and caffeinated drinks may lead to further dehydration; water and non-caffeinated herbal teas are better choices.

Natural Lubricants

Sure, you've probably heard about K-Y Jelly all your life, but if you need a lubricant for vaginal dryness, it may not be the best choice: it's a petroleum-based product that may exacerbate vaginal dryness and cause yeast infections in the long term. Using a Membrasin® sea buckthorn supplement or a natural oil such as vitamin E oil, coconut oil, or sweet almond oil might be helpful. AH! YES, a brand of lubricant gel that comes in both water- and oil-based versions, is an organic product that's worth a try (see chapter 4).

Estrogen Cream

Vaginal dryness is one condition for which hormone treatment may be a good short-term choice. A prescription hormone cream may be used to relieve your vaginal problems while you wait for more natural remedies to take effect. Estrogen cream, applied topically to the vagina, doesn't pass through the liver and therefore doesn't have the systemic effects of oral HRT.

Laser Therapy

Laser therapy, known as vaginal erbium, is now helping women to restore their vaginal tissues as well as helping to relieve stress incontinence by restoring collagen fibers that have deteriorated. New laser therapies like MonaLisa Touch claim to regenerate and heal vaginal tissues so that sex is once again comfortable. Powerful heating and microablation is applied to layers of vaginal tissue. This is a bit like the stippling effect on the peel of an orange. The technique is believed to stimulate collagen regeneration and rejuvenate the elastin fibers and blood supply to the area, which also restores lubrication and the pH in the vagina. This approach has also been shown to help reduce vaginal laxity and tighten pelvic muscles following pelvic organ prolapse.

Women who had three treatments over three months reported a significant decrease of both vaginal dryness and discomfort during sex, as well as a reduction in stress incontinence. The effects were rapid and long-lasting, persisting up to the twenty-fourth week of the observation period. Most companies suggest that women have an annual top-up treatment to maintain the benefits. This therapy may offer a promising alternative to estrogen creams (the treatment currently recommended by most doctors).

Natural Supplements and Remedies for Vaginal Dryness

Sea buckthorn oil: Supplements containing extracts from the sea buckthorn berry, such as Membrasin® Vitality Pearls (Omega 7 SBA24 in the UK), have been shown to help maintain the health and integrity of the mucous membranes in the vagina and may therefore benefit women with menopausal vaginal dryness. The plant is a source of omega-3, -6, -7, and -9 fatty acids, but it is especially high in membrasin, a monounsaturated oil. Membrasin provides the nutrients essential for the proper functioning and renewal of mucous membranes and may help to prevent vaginal inflammation and dryness.

Researchers in the Department of Obstetrics and Gynecology at the University Central Hospital in Turku, Finland, conducted a twelve-week study on the use of sea buckthorn oil in the treatment of chronic vaginal inflammation. The study looked at the symptoms of itching, burning, discharge, and dryness. The researchers concluded that "oral administration of sea buckthorn oil presents a promising alternative for treating chronic vaginal inflammation." Sea buckthorn oil contains the essential fatty acids alpha linoleic acid (omega-3) and linoleic acid (omega-6), as well as the monounsaturated fats oleic acid and palmitoleic acid.

Vitamin C: Vitamin C helps to maintain collagen, which gives skin its elasticity, and may therefore work in conjunction with the EFAs in sea buckthorn oil in helping to prevent and treat vaginal dryness. The vitamin C content of the oil may also help retain elasticity in the urinary tract and thus prevent leakage or stress incontinence, which is common at menopause.

Vitamin E oil: Vitamin E oil is a great natural remedy for feminine dryness. Using it together with black cohosh can also be helpful. Mix six capsules of vitamin E oil with about five teaspoons of cream of black cohosh and apply a small amount to the inside and outside of the vagina a couple of times a day.

Other Causes of Vaginal Dryness

Antidepressants: Many antidepressants cause vaginal drying. If you are taking one, check with your doctor about an alternative. New drugs on the market have addressed this issue, and while they may not completely solve the problem, they have been shown to dramatically reduce it.

Condoms, tampons, and douches: Using the wrong product can sometimes cause dryness. Try to stay away from anything with fragrance or added powders.

Scented soaps and powders: Stop using scented soaps, bubble baths, perfumes, and powders. The scent can cause irritation and aggravate dryness.

Prescription and over-the-counter drugs: Certain antibiotics, antihistamines, and decongestants can cause vaginal dryness if taken in large quantities. There are antibiotics that your doctor can prescribe that don't cause dryness. Avoiding decongestants and antihistamines, or using them only in the cold and flu season, can cut down on vaginal dryness. If you have seasonal allergies, talk to your doctor about nasal sprays as an alternative to oral antihistamines.

Chemotherapy and radiation If you experience painful intercourse due to vaginal dryness while undergoing cancer treatment, try using natural supplements to improve the dryness. Stay away from oil- or petroleum-based lubricants.

All these approaches may help you overcome vaginal dryness. Your life doesn't have to be miserable and your sex life doesn't have to end just because you're dealing with this problem. Once the dryness is alleviated, you will feel more like being sexually active.

Preventing Urinary Tract Infections

If recurrent UTIs are among the reasons you find yourself unenthusiastic about sex, there are steps you can take to prevent infection.

1.   Keep your vitamin D and magnesium levels topped up by taking supplements (see page 82). Low levels of these nutrients can predispose you to UTIs.
2.   When the passion is over, empty your bladder to help flush the bacteria out of the urethra, then wash yourself carefully with warm water and natural soap, patting yourself dry gently.
3.   After emptying your bladder, rock backward and forward a few times while sitting to eliminate any urine remaining in the bladder. This is another trick to flush out bacteria.
4.   Try taking D-mannose, which has been shown to reduce the number of bacteria that stick to the urethra (see page 79).

It Takes Two: Talking to Your Partner

When your libido is low, expecting your partner to understand what is going on, without explaining, is an easy trap to fall into and can quickly put a distance between you. The most important thing is that you both continue to communicate physically and emotionally. Take some time to explain what you are going through and ask for support.

In the 2019 survey "What Women Want," more than two-thirds of the 1,100 women my team and I surveyed said they found it really difficult to broach the subject of menopause with their partner. On the other hand, the survey we conducted of men and their relationships with their partners during menopause revealed that men often felt rejected, frustrated, and bewildered about what was happening to their significant other. That isn't surprising when women often don't understand it 100 percent themselves!

Having a heart-to-heart talk with your partner about what you're going through can make menopause a lot easier for both of you. It's best to start the conversation sooner rather than later so your partner doesn't attribute your symptoms or reactions to something else, and more important, so that you don't feel you have to go through this transition on your own.

Think about It

Before you can start the conversation, you need to get your head around what's going on with you. Which symptoms are affecting your life, and how? What are your fears and anxieties? How do you plan to get through menopause and reclaim your well-being? What do you think is going to be the outcome of the conversation?

Make a Date

Set a time, maybe even arrange a date night, and prepare what you are going to say. Be willing to admit your vulnerability and tell your partner that you've been worried about having this chat, but you believe there are solutions, especially if you can work through the issues together.

Be Open

Explain that you're starting to experience symptoms of menopause, including low mood and libido, that may affect your behavior, and it's not your partner's fault.

List It

Draw up a list of ways your partner may be able to help — for example, by helping you stick to a healthy eating plan. If they bring home tempting "treats" like caffeinated drinks, alcohol, or lots of chocolate, gently explain that these could make your symptoms worse. The same applies to any foods you may have developed sensitivities to, such as baked goods containing gluten.

Talk about Sex

Let your partner know you may need more time to get aroused, and suggest using a lubricant like Membrasin®, Omega 7 SBA24, AH! YES, or coconut oil.

Spend Time Together

However low you are feeling, make time for each other and let your partner know that they may be able to help you. It's amazing how much difference a hug or a snuggle on the sofa can make.

You may also want to try some of the following approaches to help you feel closer to one another.

Get in Touch

Treat each other to a sensual massage. Turn on some music, dim the lights, and start gently touching each other. Essential oils, such as jasmine, rose, ylang ylang, clary sage, or sandalwood may heighten your experience.

Experiment

If penetration is really painful, explore other ways of giving each other pleasure. Go back to your courting days and indulge in plenty of foreplay. And there is no need to shy away from using a lubricant. Rather than feeling that your cup is half full, consider oral sex as a source of pleasure.

Say it with Flowers

A dose of Bach Flower Remedies may help bring back that loving feeling. Wild rose is believed to renew interest in life and boost vitality, while olive is thought to have revitalizing properties. Larch is the one to go for if you have lost confidence in your ability to make love.

Relationship Survey

In 2018, my team and I conducted a survey of 684 women to investigate the effect of menopause on intimate relationships. The survey revealed overwhelming misery at menopause.

Although many women were interested in being sexually active — 42 percent of respondents said they used sex toys, and 31 percent watched sexy movies — 91 percent of the women in this survey felt their relationships were strained by menopause, and 79 percent reported difficulty reaching orgasm. Ninety-three percent of the respondents reported a loss of libido; 80 percent reported a lack of sensation during intercourse; 76 percent suffered with vaginal dryness; and 64 percent experienced pain on intercourse. (Thirty-five percent of those who used sex toys even experienced pain using the toy.)

Ninety-six percent of the women also reported experiencing fatigue, 91 percent experienced mood swings, and 90 percent reported trouble sleeping during menopause. Seventy percent said they would like more sex if it wasn't painful.

Hormone replacement therapy appeared to have little effect on loss of libido. Thirty-one percent of respondents had taken HRT, and 18 percent of respondents were currently taking it. Of the women who had taken HRT at some point, 64 percent reported that their libido remained suppressed or that it declined further with HRT. Fifty-four percent said problems with lack of sexual sensation remained the same or got worse.

Our survey of men in 2017 revealed that 83 percent felt rejected, saddened, or bewildered by the change in their partner. Sixty-five percent said they were no longer having a physical relationship, and 61 percent believed they could get back the girl they married!

Helen's Story

Helen, a nurse, was a past PMS client of mine who returned for help with her menopause at the age of forty-five, two weeks after having a radical hysterectomy.

After my hysterectomy I began having hot flashes and couldn't get back to sleep in the night. My doctor prescribed antidepressants, but they only wiped out what was left of my flagging libido. I didn't want to take the HRT that was prescribed by my gynecologist post-op, as HRT had such an adverse effect on my mother. My vagina was dry and itchy. I had regular chocolate cravings and migraine headaches. I was diagnosed with chronic fatigue syndrome when I was forty, but with hindsight, I think that was the start of my perimenopause.

I successfully consulted Maryon for help with my PMS a number of years ago, so I decided to ask for her help with my menopause. I followed her wise recommendations and within weeks was feeling much calmer. The headaches had gone completely, and my energy had returned. By six weeks I was pretty much symptom-free. My vaginal tissues healed and my libido returned, which delighted my husband. I feel really great again. I can't believe the difference. I'm so grateful.

What the Research Says

A pilot study using FeuchtCreme, a hormone-free cream developed by Remifemin, showed lasting improvement in treating vaginal dryness. It contains a distillate of *Hamamelis virginiana* (American witch hazel). Twenty postmenopausal women used this cream once a day for seven days and reported their symptoms before use, four to eight hours after the first application, and fourteen to twenty-two hours after the last application. Up to 80 percent reported no dryness at the end of the study. Researchers concluded that the results were promising and long-acting.

A nonsurgical, nonhormonal treatment has been developed for women having difficulty having orgasms and complaining of stress incontinence. Called TTCRF (transcutaneous temperature-controlled radiofrequency), it is an emerging procedure for treating vulvovaginal laxity and related symptoms, which sometimes affect women after childbirth and at menopause. A small study showed that after TTCRF, over 90 percent of the women took half as much time to reach orgasm, and others reported a reduction in stress incontinence and vaginal tissue deterioration. Women were reportedly able to stop using vaginal estrogen creams.

A small study at Tel Aviv University showed that women taking magnesium supplements twice a day experienced a reduction in urinary incontinence symptoms and did not wake up as many times in the night to go to the bathroom. This may be because magnesium reduces bladder muscle spasms and allows the bladder to empty completely.

At this stage in our lives, sex is more about recreation than procreation, which means we should be able to have more physical fun than ever. Breaking down the taboo surrounding this very personal problem can help us access natural, scientifically proven solutions so that we and our partners can once again enjoy a fulfilling sex life.

Busting Stress

Anxieties about sex are intertwined with another common and debilitating midlife problem: stress. While a little stress in our lives can keep us on our toes, at other times, especially when we are trying to balance family, children, relationships, work, and finances as well as menopause, even the smallest amount of stress can tip the scales and leave us in a very negative place.

Stress is on the increase, and its physical effects are being felt. According to a global Gallup poll conducted on 150,000 people in 2018, Americans are among the most stressed-out people in the world. The reports of feeling more stress and worry were at the highest level seen in Gallup's regular poll for a decade. An American study published in the *Journal of Sports Medicine* in 2018 showed a relationship between gut upsets and life stress and anxiety in a group of runners. A survey of over a thousand Australian midwives, with an average age of forty-six, showed that over two-thirds of them were suffering from burnout. Around 20 percent of the women reported moderate to extreme levels of depression, and anxiety levels were high as well.

There is no doubt that stress makes menopause symptoms far worse. Rushing around, being under pressure to meet a deadline or attend a meeting, worrying whether you'll melt in public, or dealing with a difficult family situation can bring on a hot flash. In addition, your normal coping skills may be significantly reduced in menopause because of poor sleep disrupted by night sweats, among other factors.

Stress causes hormonal changes in the body, including elevated levels of cortisol, a steroid hormone produced in the adrenal glands. Cortisol production is a component of the fight-or-flight mechanism in our autonomic nervous system that revs up our body in response to a threat. In the long term, elevated cortisol levels can cause many symptoms similar to menopause symptoms, including brain fog, fatigue, anxiety, low mood, even depression, an increase in belly fat, and, in extreme cases, chronic inflammation.

Women Feeling Stressed: Statistics

In a recent international study of thirteen thousand people conducted by Cigna, 84 percent of respondents believed they suffered from stress, with 13 percent of them describing themselves unable to manage. And that was before COVID-19 hit us!

The survey found that women were more stressed than men, many of them juggling both work and family life. They didn't feel supported at work, with only half saying their employers had any well-being packages in place.

According to *Forbes,* many women were already at breaking point because of workplace stress. But home life can also be a significant cause of stress. In *Prevention* magazine's latest survey in 2019, conducted in conjunction with GCI Health, 54 percent of American women described themselves as more stressed than their partner. Among many choices of major stressors, "family" and "household clutter or projects" were consistently listed as the top two. Backing that up, a 2010 study from UCLA found that women who described their homes with words like "mess" and "chaotic" didn't see their cortisol levels drop at the end of the day as most men did.

A Kaiser Family Foundation study featured on *Good Morning America* agrees that women are more stressed than men and that this is likely to have a negative impact on their mental health. Even women who work outside the home tend to do a greater share of caregiving tasks than their male partners and more of the household chores. In addition, a Harvard University study has found that women do the bulk of the cognitive labor for household tasks, including anticipating and monitoring what needs to be done.

Quiz: How Stressed Are You?

- Are you tired all the time?
- Do you have trouble sleeping or wake up in the middle of the night?
- Do you crave sugary foods?
- Do you keep bursting into tears?
- Do you get frequent headaches?
- Do you find it hard to make up your mind?
- Do you get butterflies in your stomach?
- Do you feel anxious or on edge for no special reason?
- Do you have you emotional problems?
- Are your family relationships strained?
- Are you forgetful?
- Is your digestive system upset?
- Is your appetite reduced?
- Do you sometimes feel it's all too much?
- Do you find it difficult to communicate with people?
- Do you have too little time for yourself?
- Have your symptoms worsened as a result of recent events?

If you answered yes to more than three of these questions, the chances are you're suffering from stress overload. If you scored more than six, you need to take some action to reduce your stress levels and protect your health. Remember to enter your score on your Natural Menopause Solution worksheet.

Action Plan

At midlife, probably more so than at any other time in our lives so far, it's important for us to have strategies in place to minimize stress. First we need to identify any obvious triggers and eliminate them or try to deal with them as best we can. Find some quiet time to think about and make a list of the things that cause you stress. Once you have identified these, you get can started on some simple stress-management techniques.

Top Stress Busters

In troubled and unpredictable times it's understandable to not want to get out of bed in the morning. We all have choices when we awaken. We can drift through the day feeling negative and scared, listening to every news report, or we can learn to live in the moment, focusing on making it a special day, filled with actions that will help others and, at the same time, make us feel happy. Our happiness is largely in our own hands.

Breathe and be mindful: Staying in the moment, refusing to listen to those negative voices in your head, is key to staying sane and happy. There are great TED talks on the benefits of breathing and mindfulness, and books like *All Is Well*, by Louise Hay and Mona Lisa Schulz, provide affirmations you can use while doing some mindful breathing to help calm you down.

> Within the first few weeks of being on Maryon's Natural Menopause Solution I began losing weight immediately, brain fog disappeared a bit later, and sleep got gradually better. The difference for me is like the difference between night and day.
>
> — Barbara Gustafson

Organize your time: Define your priorities so you can use your time and energy efficiently. Make a realistic to-do list at the beginning of each day. Learn to say no: you don't have to agree to everything people ask you to do. If you haven't got a structured work life at present, make yourself a timetable full of activities and stick to it. You'll feel less stressed by getting out of bed and engaging in productive activity than by watching TV, surfing the internet, and eating junk food.

Embrace family time: For many people, a silver lining of the strict COVID-19 restrictions on work, school, and travel was a slowing down of the hectic pace of our lives. With the world on pause, we had an opportunity to embrace family living and derive joy from the small things that happen when we have the time to be loving and giving. For those who had the misfortune to be separated from family, staying in touch virtually helped to keep the feel-good hormones flowing. Regardless of what the future has in store, we can keep in mind the benefits of connecting with our loved ones and make time for it to happen.

Find inner joy: In *The Book of Joy*, the Dalai Lama and Bishop Desmond Tutu observe that acts of kindness are the best way to guarantee your own happiness and experience joy. I highly recommend this book: reading it was a life-changing experience for me.

Appreciate each day: As well as doing random acts of kindness, take time to nurture yourself. Make a point of appreciating the beauty of nature each day. If you can't get outdoors, capture some gorgeous images on a Pinterest board.

Make a gratitude list: Giving some serious thought to all that you have to be grateful for can help keep things in perspective. We often forget that just being able to see beauty, hear wonderful sounds, and smell delicious food are all blessings. Think about people and places you are grateful for. Keep adding to your list and look at it regularly, especially when you are feeling down.

Relax: Make time for relaxation on a daily basis, whether it's yoga, meditation, soaking in a warm bath, listening to music, dancing to your favorite music, going for a walk, or reading a book. There are a number of apps that can help you to chill out and lower your level of stress hormones. Good options include Pzizz and Headspace (see chapter 4).

Eat well: Include plenty of magnesium-rich foods in your diet, such as spinach, Brazil nuts, and walnuts. Magnesium supports the nervous system and has calming properties.

Resist the temptation to reach for "comfort" foods such as chocolate, cakes, cookies, soft drinks, alcohol, tea, and coffee. Sugary foods can cause a spike and then a drop in blood sugar levels, causing a downturn in mood. In addition, these foods may interfere with your body's ability to absorb vitamins and minerals, often making you feel even worse. Eating foods that are naturally sweet, such as fresh or dried fruit, as well as nuts and seeds, is a much healthier option. And go for rooibos tea or relaxing herbal teas rather than black tea or coffee, which are high in caffeine and can make you jittery. See page 68 for tips on dealing with cravings.

Boost your nutrient levels: Take a strong multivitamin and mineral supplement like Gynovite Plus or Fema 45+ daily. Adaptogenic herbs, including rhodiola, ashwagandha, and holy basil, can help your body to deal with stress (but check with your doctor first for compatibility with any medications you are taking).

Get moving: One of the best stress busters is physical exercise. Regular activity helps speed up the metabolism and encourages the release of endorphins, the body's own feel-good hormones.

Stay in touch: Stay connected with loved ones and friends. Even if we can't visit in person, most of us have access to phone or computer apps that make it easy to stay in contact. Since the COVID-19 pandemic began, I've been hearing that people are connecting with distant friends and family in a way they haven't for years. Loneliness is a significant cause of depression; reaching out to others can help everyone.

Declutter: Getting rid of things we no longer want or need feels cleansing and therapeutic, opening up mental and physical space. Take one drawer or closet at a time. If you can't face doing it alone, connect with a friend on WhatsApp to do it together. If your area is in lockdown, you may not be able to get your clutter out of the house, but you can create clutter boxes that can be stored and then donated when thrift shops and recycling centers reopen.

Make your heart sing: A rule I live by these days is to do more of the things that make my heart sing and say no to things that make my heart sink! Research shows that pursuits that make us feel good are likely to reduce our cortisol levels. This could mean watching a funny movie, laughing with friends, letting your inner child out, or having cuddles and great sex.

Sleeping Peacefully

The link between lack of sleep and mood disorders is well documented. If we get less than seven to nine hours of quality sleep each night, it can seriously affect everything from our physical well-being to our motivation and emotions. Even mild sleep deprivation can make us more irritable and leave us feeling depressed, sad, and depleted. People suffering with insomnia have been shown to be ten times more likely to experience depression and seventeen times more likely to suffer with anxiety. So lack of sleep can affect our relationships both at home and at work, which in itself can be depressing.

I'm sleeping better and no longer need a sleeping pill, and if I do wake in the night, I get straight back to sleep now. I've lost weight, I'm able to concentrate and listen and am no longer forgetful. This program has truly been a life changer for me.

— Lisa Finn

Problems getting to sleep and staying asleep become more common as we approach and go through menopause. In fact, insomnia is one of the most common menopause symptoms. And given what's happening to the body, it's not surprising. In addition to night sweats, which disrupt sleep, we're experiencing a drop in the sleep-promoting hormone progesterone.

It's a vicious circle, for the more elusive sleep becomes, the more likely we are to feel anxious, depressed, irritable, and exhausted. Before we know it we can get caught up in a whirlwind of anxious thoughts, which lead to more bad sleep.

Low levels of nutrients can cause restless leg syndrome, an uncomfortable sensation that triggers an often uncontrollable urge to move your feet and legs. It can be addressed by topping up on vitamin D, iron, folate, magnesium, and calcium. It usually takes only a few weeks for this symptom to disappear once the nutrients start to take effect.

Action Plan

Fortunately, we can find ways to help us sleep peacefully again without resorting to medication. Changes in our environment, habits, and diet can promote more restful sleep.

Set the Scene

Your bedroom should be a sanctuary for sleep, with all tablets, mobile phones, e-readers, and laptops left outside the door. The glare from these screens emits a blue light that disrupts the function of the pineal gland in the brain, blocking production of the sleep-inducing hormone melatonin, so using electronic devices just before bedtime can interfere with good sleep. It's not just screen glare, though. The light from digital clocks, radios, security sensors, and charger units can all disrupt sleep patterns. Remove them, shroud them with a dark cloth, or stick a piece of black tape over them.

Keep your bedroom dark. Darkness triggers the production of melatonin, while light prevents its release or shuts it off. Even the tiniest chink of light can trick your brain into thinking it's morning and waking you. Go for tight-fitting blackout curtains or blinds in your bedroom.

Eat Wisely

What you eat and when can have a profound effect on how well you sleep. For example, eating dinner late and going to bed on a full stomach can lead to a disrupted night. For about two hours after eating a meal, the digestive process is hard at work, meaning that the body cannot rest.

To produce melatonin, the body needs the neurotransmitting chemical serotonin. To produce serotonin, in turn, the body requires a supply of the amino acid tryptophan, which is found in turkey, chicken, eggs, beans, lentils, fish, soy, oats, and milk. Try to include some of these foods in your evening meal. A handful of edamame beans and a small glass of slightly warmed soy milk an hour before bedtime can also help increase serotonin levels.

If you've already increased your intake of isoflavones in keeping with the recommendations of this program, you may already be on the way to better sleep. A Japanese study showed that low-dose isoflavones can be effective in relieving depression and insomnia linked to menopause. Ninety women received an ultra-low dose (12.5 mg/day) or a low dose (25 mg/day) of the isoflavone aglycone or a placebo for eight weeks. Significant improvement in depressive and insomnia symptoms was observed in those on the low-dose isoflavone supplement.

Keep to a Bedtime Routine

Try to go to bed at the same time each night and wake at the same time each morning — even on weekends. Our circadian rhythms (our body's internal clock) are individual, so it is important to work out your own optimal sleep and wake times. Shift workers will find this more difficult, as will those who are disturbed by the schedules of other family members. When you are reestablishing peaceful sleep, you will need to find a peaceful space and ask for support.

Wind Down Gently

Get into a relaxing bedtime routine: for example, a warm bath with a few drops of calming essential oils, such as lavender, chamomile, or lemongrass ; a soothing cup of warm soy milk, or chamomile or valerian tea; or a quiet chat with your partner. Or pour magnesium salts into that bath to help relax your body and ease aching muscles.

Avoid watching or reading anything too stimulating in the evening, as it may keep you awake. Instead, listen to some soothing music, do some sewing or knitting, quietly read from the printed page, or do some gentle upper-body stretches or light yoga to loosen up tight muscles and help you relax. Resist the temptation to just flop into bed.

Keep It Cool

Wear loose-fitting nightwear made from natural fabrics such as silk, cotton, and wool. Open the windows and keep your bedroom as cool as you can. Between 58 and 70 degrees Fahrenheit (about 15–21 degrees Celsius) is thought to be an ideal bedroom temperature, although I think that's pretty cool. Use layers of lightweight bedding that you can adjust according to how hot you feel, and keep some cooling wipes beside your bed within easy reach in case of hot flashes. Don't sleep with an electric blanket on, as this disturbs sleep patterns by increasing core body temperature, not to mention exacerbating hot flashes.

Stay Calm

Fretting about not being able to sleep is the one thing guaranteed to stop you entering the land of Nod. Whether it's counting sheep, reading a book, or meditating before bed, do something that soothes you and prevents you from worrying about being awake. If you do find yourself waking up in the middle of the night, consider downloading the Pzizz Sleep app, developed by neuroscientists, to help you get back to sleep.

Be Mindful

Mindfulness (see page 91) has been found to help sleep. Focusing on your breathing is a key technique. Simply concentrate on breathing naturally in and out. Don't force yourself to breathe deeply; just be aware of your breath. If thoughts, emotions, or awareness of your surroundings starts to intrude, simply bring your mind back to your breathing, without judgment.

Supplement It

Sleeping pills often just relieve the symptoms of insomnia rather than the causes, and they can cause side effects and dependency. A better alternative is to consider natural remedies such as passionflower, L-theanine, and valerian, which have been found to help promote healthy sleep patterns and relieve anxiety, without the risk of side effects such as a foggy brain on waking.

Valerian: *Valeriana officinalis*, sometimes described as nature's tranquilizer, grows wild in North America and Europe, although it is also cultivated for medicinal purposes. It has been taken for centuries to treat nervous anxiety, reduce muscle tension, and relieve mild insomnia. Valerian contains several unique substances, such as valerenic acid and valeranon, that relax the muscles and central nervous system and are particularly effective in treating stress and anxiety. It's an herb to consider for the relief of anxiety and panic attacks.

On its own or as an ingredient in herbal sleep remedies, valerian can relieve insomnia and improve sleep quality by calming the brain and body, rather than inducing sleep directly, so that sleep can occur naturally. It is nonaddictive and has few side effects compared to more conventional sleep remedies.

For insomnia, take 1,600 mg of valerian a day, or four 400 mg tablets. To reduce stress, take up to 2,400 mg a day (6 tablets), evenly distributed throughout the day. It may take several weeks before you see an improvement in mild insomnia. Because valerian enhances the action of sleep-enhancing drugs, it should not be taken in conjunction with sleeping pills or tranquilizers, although it can be combined with other herbs.

Passionflower: *Passiflora incarnata* is a climbing shrub native to South America and Europe. Passionflower was valued by Native Americans for its ability to heal bruises and wounds. Other herbal practitioners value the plant for its calming, sedative, and pain-relieving effects, and it has been used over the years to treat anxiety, fatigue, insomnia, and muscle spasms. It can also help soothe period pains and tension headaches.

Passionflower is often used for insomnia, especially when the root cause is nervousness. Like valerian, with which it is often combined, it is popular for its gentle, nonaddictive sedative properties. Take 0.5–1 g of dried extract three times a day or 1.4 mL tincture three to four times a day.

L-theanine: L-theanine is an amino acid found in tea leaves. It is thought to ease anxiety and promote more peaceful sleep. Since tea contains caffeine, it's better to take this substance in supplement form if you're experiencing sleep problems. The body responds relatively quickly when a dose is taken. The recommended dose is 200 mg per day or night, ideally taken with food. If you take medication for hypertension you will need to get your blood pressure checked regularly, because L-theanine has been shown to lower blood pressure.

Keep Moving

Study after study shows that regular exercise promotes longer, better sleep. Sleep experts used to advise avoiding evening exercise, but they now suggest listening to your own body clock. If you're a night owl, evening exercise may suit you better. Exercising an hour and a half before bedtime has been linked with more deep sleep and less of the lighter REM (dreaming) sleep.

To promote sleep, aim for thirty minutes a day of aerobic exercise like walking, swimming, cycling, or dancing, plus a couple of sessions of resistance exercise, such as a weight workout, each week (see chapter 4). Yoga, tai chi, Pilates, and other mind-body activities also help relieve anxiety and can ease you into sleep.

Worry Not

Anxiety is the biggest enemy of sleep. If you're worried about anything — work, finances, health, family — write down your thoughts or make a to-do list before you go to bed. It really helps to clear the mind, making it easier to sleep. And if you do wake up, don't look at the clock: cover it up, hide it, or turn it around.

Beware the Nightcap

That late-night comfort drink may relax you and make you sleepy, but once your body has metabolized the alcohol, chances are you'll be wide awake at 4 a.m. Even limiting yourself to the healthy drinking guideline of one drink a day for women will wash away important nutrients and bring on hot flashes and night sweats as you journey through menopause. Some women feel a hot flash coming on after just a sip of wine or a hot drink. If you drink, limit your intake to one glass of wine twice a week in the evening, preferably with a meal and at least two hours before bedtime. Also avoid caffeinated drinks: women metabolize caffeine more slowly at midlife. Even decaffeinated drinks can trigger a hot flash.

Watch Fluid Intake

If you find yourself waking up and having to go to the bathroom more often than you used to, which is a common midlife symptom, try not to drink any fluids, other than sips, within a couple of hours of bedtime. Reduce your evening consumption of hot drinks and diuretics such as alcohol and caffeine. Before going to bed, go to the bathroom twice within five minutes to empty your bladder completely.

Beat the Grunts

A snoring partner can prevent peaceful sleep, so consider investing in some soft foam earplugs. Alternatively, suggest they sleep on their side, lose weight if they need to, and avoid smoking or drinking within five hours of bedtime. A persistent snorer should consider getting tested for sleep apnea — and that includes you if you're experiencing problems. Professional singers rarely snore, possibly because singing exercises the throat muscles, so you could also suggest that your partner join a choir! Orgasms have also been shown to promote restful sleep. (Even though you may not be feeling super sexy at the moment, I thought it was worth mentioning, as you will eventually get your sexy back.)

Julie's Story

Julie, who helps administer my course, had no idea that her symptoms were related to perimenopause until she heard me talking to other women. She'd had debilitating insomnia for two years.

By the time I reached fifty, I felt exhausted all the time. I hadn't slept for more than two hours at a stretch for two years and didn't know why. It wasn't until I met Maryon that I realized I was perimenopausal, as I had none of what I believed to be the classic symptoms, such as hot flashes. It was never suggested by anyone. My limbs ached constantly, and I just thought I was getting old.

Maryon was setting up a course, and I was hired as the course administrator. When I heard that insomnia was a common perimenopause symptom, I realized that I had reached that life stage. So as well as managing the course, I joined as a participant.

Within four weeks of starting Maryon's Six-Week Natural Menopause Solution, I began to sleep again. I couldn't believe it. I no longer have brain fog or aching limbs and have taken up boxing to keep fit. I feel younger, sexier, and more confident, and people tell me I look younger than I did ten years ago.

Chapter 6 marks the final week of the Six-Week Natural Menopause Solution. It focuses on restoring both short and long-term memory and mental clarity, banishing hair loss, staying wise and positive — and helping you to shape the rest of your recovery journey and enhance your long-term health.

Chapter 6

WEEK SIX

Memory, Healthy Hair, and Staying Positive

Boosting Memory and Reclaiming Mental Clarity

Feeling like you are losing your memory at midlife can be very frightening, especially if you think it's permanent. Many women secretly wonder if these "senior moments" are the beginning of early-onset Alzheimer's disease or dementia and are truly freaked out.

If you forget what you are saying in midsentence, what you went into a room for, or where you put your car keys, you are not alone. It's one of the commonest symptoms of menopause. You are not losing your marbles. We all start to forget things as we age, say the experts. Among a group of people asked to memorize a list of seventy-five words read out five times, the average eighteen-year-old scored 54, a forty-five-year-old scored 47, and a sixty-five-year-old scored just 37.

No one knows the reason for sure, but it's thought most memory problems at this time of life are due to a combination of poor concentration, lack of motivation, tiredness, anxiety, and stress, rather than loss of brain cells. Feeling fuzzy-headed is also thought to be related to the hormonal ups and downs associated with menopause. Nutrition plays a role too: the brain goes into economy mode when it has a low level of nutrients, which makes thinking less clear. And as we grow older, our circulation slows down, and less oxygen reaches our brain cells.

Some parts of the brain particularly involved with verbal memory are rich in estrogen receptors, so there could be a physiological link between hormonal status and brain function, as suggested by research undertaken by Sandra File at Guy's Hospital in London.

Like our muscles, our brain needs exercise in order to function optimally. Many of us don't stretch our brains as much as we could. Following a nutrient-dense and phytoestrogen-rich diet, leading an active lifestyle, not smoking, limiting alcohol intake, and keeping your brain well exercised can all help to keep you sharp.

Food for Thought

The brain is dependent on glucose, essential fats, and phospholipids. Several B vitamins are also essential for memory and mental performance. Zinc and magnesium are necessary for neurotransmitter function. It follows that including certain nutrients in your diet can help boost your concentration, attention span, and both short- and long-term memory. Research also suggests that brain-boosting supplements can help improve your memory. Indeed more than three hundred medical studies have been published on memory, most indicating the benefits of taking daily supplements.

An extract made from the leaves of *Gingko biloba,* commonly known as gingko or the Chinese maidenhair tree, has gained recognition over the past thirty years for helping restore vascular function and memory. Ginkgo improves circulation, which in turn increases blood flow, carrying more nutrients and oxygen to the brain. This helps restore short-term and long-term memory, helping you to think more clearly and concentrate better.

Foods rich in the antioxidant vitamins A, C, and E help mop up free radicals, the rogue molecules that can cause cell damage in the body, including the brain. Good sources include richly colored fruits and vegetables, such as bananas, red peppers, spinach, and oranges.

Oily fish is rich in omega-3 essential fatty acids and folate, which are vital for the functioning of the brain and nervous system. Good sources include sardines, salmon, herring, anchovies, and mackerel.

Eating soy has been shown to improve memory in menopausal women. These research findings have led to speculation that soy may also help maintain cognitive function in older women and reduce the risk of Alzheimer's disease.

Quiz: How Sharp Is Your Brain?

- Do you ever forget what you went upstairs for?
- Do you have trouble remembering telephone numbers?

- Do you find it hard to concentrate?
- Do you forget a person's name the moment after you've been introduced?
- Are you prone to absentminded acts, such as putting milk in the cupboard instead of the refrigerator?
- Have you ever missed an appointment because you forgot it?
- Do you have to write arrangements down the minute you make them for fear of forgetting them?
- Have you ever forgotten the name of someone you know well?
- Do you frequently lose your car keys?
- Have you ever forgotten what you were saying midsentence?
- Have you ever gone to mention something important to someone, but gone completely blank?
- Have you ever put something in the oven and forgotten to take it out?
- Have you ever said you would do something for someone, but completely forgotten to do it?

If you answered yes to more than three questions, it's time to try some memory-boosting foods and supplements, as well as doing some mental exercises.

Staying Sharp

Many studies show that stimulation is the key to good memory and that people who take part in lots of different types of mental activity have better powers of recall. The more active your brain is, the better your memory is likely to be, and the more different ways you use your mind, the easier you'll find it to remember things. It's all to do with being active, rather than passive: whether you actively concentrate and focus on things or whether you just let them wash over you. Try the following exercises to sharpen your mental faculties:

- Do a mental exercise every day — a crossword, sudoku, word search, or quiz. If you don't know the solution, look it up, then try to remember it the next day.
- When doing your finances, ditch the calculator and use your brain instead.
- Take up new activities — gardening, knitting, or anything involving physical coordination.

- Memorize your shopping list before going to the store.
- Engage in games that stretch your brain, such as chess or bridge.

Our memory allows us to learn new things and store millions of facts and figures in words, sound, and picture form. Even if we fed information into our brain every second of our lives, it would find room to store all we needed to recall. We rely on the information retained in our memory to respond to environmental and social stimulation every day of our lives.

What the Research Says

As we age, many nutrients may be in short supply. Deficiencies of the B vitamins (including B12) and vitamin D are associated with cognitive impairment as well as depression.

Vitamin E and other antioxidants may be important in maintaining blood flow to the brain and the central nervous system. One study showed that patients with early signs of dementia improved after being given high doses of vitamin E.

There is recent scientific evidence that soy isoflavones, in dietary or supplement form, can help with cognitive and psychological symptoms around menopause. There is a high concentration of estrogen receptors in the hippocampus — the part of the brain responsible for memory and learning — that these molecules might bind to. An analysis of ten randomized, placebo-controlled clinical trials of isoflavone supplement use involving more than one thousand women showed that isoflavones were associated with a significant improvement in cognitive function and visual memory. The effect was greatest among women under the age of sixty and, perhaps surprisingly, for shorter periods of treatment. The researchers suggest there could be an important "window of opportunity" during which supplementation and dietary changes should be started for maximum benefit.

The Women's Isoflavone Soy Health Trial looked at the cognitive effects of long-term intake of soy isoflavones at levels comparable to those of traditional Asian diets. This trial was longer and larger than previous trials of soy isoflavones for cognition. Women took a daily dose of 25 grams of isoflavone-rich soy protein or placebo for two and a half years. The soy protein supplement contained 52 mg genistein, 36 mg daidzein, and 3 mg glycitein. The most pronounced improvement was a strong increase in the capacity to remember faces.

Andrea's Story

Andrea is an executive and soul mastery leadership coach in the San Francisco Bay Area. She was living a healthy lifestyle when we were introduced but was still suffering with menopause symptoms.

My goal was to enter menopause as fit and healthy as I could be so as to meet it head-on. I worked out regularly, meditated, and ate "clean," healthy, organic foods too. I figured if I did all this, I was bound to be okay. Right?

And I was okay until the year I turned fifty-one, when night sweats seemed to hit me out of nowhere. It was like a light switch. I'd go to bed, get maybe one to two hours of sleep, and then wake two, three, sometimes even four times during the night, completely drenched in sweat. It was miserable. Chronic sleepless nights led to days spent in a brain fog. I was so tired. It was hard to concentrate, to think clearly, to focus. I worried about making mistakes in my work, forgetting simple little things. It was mentally and emotionally debilitating. I was miserable. This went on for about three to four weeks, and I knew I had to do something about it. I couldn't live this way. I needed help.

Luckily at the time I was working with a business coach who, upon hearing of my misery and knowing my desire to use a natural approach to mitigating menopause, recommended Maryon Stewart to me. I checked out her website, liked what I saw, and signed up for her complimentary master class. After that I immediately signed up for her six-week virtual menopause course.

I'm so glad I did and am eternally grateful to Maryon and the work she does in the world. Maryon uses a multipronged, science-backed approach in her program. It includes areas I already had a head start in (things like meditation, exercise, and healthy eating) but included areas that I didn't have knowledge in as they pertain to menopause, including supplements tailored to your symptoms, and recommendations of natural foods to help replace estrogen.

After taking supplements and including naturally occurring estrogen regularly in my diet, I began to feel so much better. By the end of the six weeks, the severe night sweats were almost gone, and I was sleeping much better. Heaven!

Two years in, I now know my body in this stage of life so much better. Symptoms are for the most part gone. If they do arise, they aren't too bad, and I know what lifestyle habits I've slipped into that have caused them. I also know what to do to get back on track.

I'm also glad to know how to fend off osteoporosis. While I rate above average in bone density for my age, I've started to see it decline, as it does after menopause, and feel I'm doing everything naturally to keep my bones strong.

Menopause, and applying Maryon's advice, is a learning process, so give yourself time to practice, because you are worth it. I'm lucky in that I have a very supportive husband and family that I can talk to, and that I didn't waste much time (one month) to address my issues when they got bad. I knew I wanted to feel well.

What saddens me about this whole process is how few women talk openly about menopause. I spoke with friends openly, and when I did, they poured out their tales of woe. But so many women put up with the symptoms and resort to nonnatural methods, or opt for the quick fixes that ultimately are more harmful than good — when they don't have to.

> If we could give every individual the right amount of nourishment and exercise, not too little and not too much, we would have found the safest way to health.
>
> — Hippocrates

Reducing Hair Loss

Hair loss is often associated with men, but in fact millions of women also experience it, particularly at the time of menopause, when estrogen and progesterone levels are falling.

Some women find their hair thins all over, while others get what's known as alopecia areata, which results in patches of complete hair loss. Generalized, often mild, scalp hair loss can also accompany diseases of the scalp, such as psoriasis and eczema.

A large proportion of women reporting hair loss have low levels of ferritin, a blood protein that contains iron. This is common among women who have heavy periods or experience flooding during perimenopause, which causes a gradual depletion of iron stores. Vegetarians are more likely to have low serum ferritin levels than meat eaters.

See your doctor to investigate possible other causes, such as:

- An underactive thyroid gland or other hormonal disturbance
- A fever or any severe illness
- A side effect of medication
- Chronic iron deficiency

Ways to Combat Thinning Hair

Eat a Nutritious Diet

Eat iron-rich foods such as liver, beef, lamb, almonds, lentils, Brazil nuts, eggs, spinach, muesli, fortified cereals. and whole grains. Many of these foods are also rich in vitamin B7 (biotin), which is essential for healthy hair.

Brazil nuts are also one of the best sources of the trace mineral selenium, which is needed for the production of thyroid hormones. Zinc, found in beef, lamb, Brazil nuts, peanuts, turkey, wholegrain bread, cheddar cheese, prawns, and oysters, is also important.

Salmon, sprats, sardines, chickpeas, chicken, flaxseeds, sesame seeds, walnuts, red meat, and quinoa contain a range of the essential nutrients, including zinc, essential fats and iron, that can help promote hair growth.

Soy-based foods and drinks provide a rich source of iron as well as being a great source of naturally occurring estrogen.

Avoid black tea, as it contains tannin, which binds with iron and inhibits its absorption.

Take Supplements

Take an iron supplement if you are anemic or if your hemoglobin level is toward the low end of normal (11.0–12.5 mg/dL). Don't overdo it, as iron can be harmful in excessive doses. A small supplement, such as one tablet of ferrous sulfate taken daily with fruit juice, is safe and should correct any mild deficiency. You will need to take it for six months, as recovery is slow.

Vitamin C works synergistically with iron, enhancing its absorption. Take a supplement of at least 1,000 mg a day.

It's useful to take supplements including omega-3 and omega-6 essential fatty acids, antioxidants, zinc, calcium pantothenate (vitamin B5), and biotin. Specialized products like Florisene and Nourkrin have been shown to help prevent hair shedding. Supplements can be ordered from maryonstewart.com/shop.

Use Appropriate Hair-Care Products

Use a gentle shampoo and conditioner that doesn't contain any harmful chemicals, including sodium lauryl sulfate (SLS), parabens, triclosan, and polyethylene glycol (aka PEG). Examples include SheaMoisture Jamaican Black Castor Oil shampoo, which contains shea butter, peppermint, and apple cider vinegar and claims to strengthen and restore hair; and SheaMoisture 100% Virgin Coconut Oil Daily Hydration Conditioner with coconut milk and acacia senegal, known for its fiber-repairing and hydration qualities. Both products are sulfate-free and safe for colored hair.

The Biokera range of hair products is claimed to help calm an irritated scalp and thicken hair. Biokera Scalp Therapy Intensive Serum contains components that claim to stimulate cellular metabolism and promote hair growth.

What the Research Says

A randomized study carried out in France on 120 women found that hair density significantly improved over a six-month period when women took a supplement containing omega-3 and omega-6 EFAs, plus other antioxidant nutrients. Reductions in perceived hair loss were also noted.

A recent review on alopecia areata noted a deficiency of folate, vitamin D, and zinc in sufferers. A small number of studies have suggested that vitamin A can mitigate the effects of the disease.

Staying Wise and Positive: Secrets to Feeling Amazing Forever

Many of us have negative thoughts and low self-esteem at the time of menopause. And that's not surprising if we are suffering from a lack of sleep, hot flashes, night sweats, bulging waistlines, and low libido. Instead of enjoying the sense that others find us attractive, we may begin to feel invisible. The feeling of unattractiveness is not helped by the attitude of many men that we are now just "women of a certain age."

What matters most is how you feel about yourself. If you feel well and take care of your health, your well-being will be reflected in your skin, hair, and nails. There will be a spring in your step and you will glow from the inside. If you have lost your sparkle, it's possible to reframe your attitudes and habits and get back to being your old self or even better. Amy Ahlers and Christine Arylo's book *Reform Your Inner Mean Girl* provides great tools to quiet your inner bully.

At the time of menopause we don't have to contend with just our own negative views; we also often lack support from medical professionals. It's not that they are negative people — far from it, they are members of the caring profession — but they often admit to being inadequately informed. We know from the 2019 Mayo Clinic survey of doctors and gynecologists that only 7 percent of them felt adequately educated to help women going through menopause. As a result, they can't identify the tools you need to help you dig yourself out of the hole.

In addition, support, or lack of it, from healthcare providers makes a difference to our well-being. Numerous reputable studies have shown that the attitude of doctors and their teams is directly related to patients' health outcomes. If you are told by your doctor that your symptoms are "all part of the aging process" or that "you'll have to live with it," you are much more likely to believe that you will remain unwell. On the other hand, if your healthcare team has a positive, optimistic approach, you are more likely to recover. The same is true of our own outlook on things. Optimists have healthier hearts, for example, while pessimists are more likely to get sick and be depressed. Those with higher self-esteem not only have lower rates of heart disease but also have lower levels of the stress hormone cortisol.

Changing Attitudes

Our attitudes are affected in a number of ways as we enter midlife. Those effects can be broken down into the messages that come from within us and those that come from the world around us.

Attitudes toward menopause can be both positive and negative. Some women are delighted that their periods are over and are happy to grow older gracefully, while others are horrified by the process, mourning the loss of their fertility and worrying that it will be all downhill from here. Many women are affected by the ubiquitous advertising and media coverage that sends the message that young and beautiful women are much more valued in our society than older, wiser women.

In our survey of women's attitudes at the time of menopause, 80 percent of women surveyed were delighted their periods had stopped; but 40 percent were anxious and afraid of changes in their physical appearance, 37 percent felt that menopause signaled the start of old age, and 17 percent thought their partner would prefer a younger woman.

These results make depressing reading, yet most of them can be termed "crooked" thinking because, once the physical symptoms of menopause have been overcome and fatigue is no longer an issue, the midlife years can be an enormously positive phase in your life. They should be seen not so much as the end of the reproductive years but as the beginning or rebirth of a whole new you. As my sister, Sue Fisher, once said, you need to spend less time hanging around the fountain of youth and more time bathing in the waters of wisdom!

The first step to changing the way you think is to learn to love yourself for who you are and to accept the stage of life you are in. The secret is to embrace midlife, not run away from it.

Quiz: How's Your Self-Esteem?

- Do you feel unattractive?
- Do you think life as you once knew it is over?
- Do you see yourself as old?
- Do you see menopause as the beginning of the end?
- Do you think your partner (if you have one) no longer finds you attractive?
- Do you think your partner would prefer to be with a younger woman?
- If you don't have a partner, do you think you are now too old to find one?
- Do you tend to concentrate on your bad points rather than your good points?
- Do you tend to dwell on your failures rather than your achievements?
- Are you unhappy with what you have achieved in life?
- Do you sometimes doubt your ability to succeed?
- Do you see life as all downhill from now on?
- Do you wish you were young again?
- Do you think you were more attractive when you were younger?

- Do you think you are too old for good sex?
- Do you dread menopause?

If you answered yes to more than three questions, read on to learn how you can change your attitudes and start feeling good about yourself again.

Action Plan

Create Some Me Time

The key to an emotionally healthy and rewarding midlife is to examine the attitudes that affect you. Spend some time working out what your priorities and values are at this time of life. They may be very different from what they were ten years ago. Find time to get to know yourself again, as well as time to laugh and share friendships and nurture your precious sense of humor.

It is also vital to achieve a relaxed "head space." Both the physical and emotional symptoms of menopause are made significantly worse by stress, so relaxation and meditation techniques are a must. Try to find an hour each day to exercise, relax, or meditate. See page 90 for suggestions on helpful activities.

Pat Yourself on the Back

Get yourself a notebook and keep a note of your daily achievements and lifetime achievements, large or small. It is all too easy to move on to the next thing, or even the next day, without acknowledging what you have accomplished. Acknowledge your success in the workplace or at rearing amazing children into functioning adults. Again, we tend to fixate on our mistakes and things we regret. Making time to review your successes helps you build self-confidence. Read back over your notebook each week and congratulate yourself on how well you are doing.

Engage in Mutual Support

The rewards that come from helping make other people's lives more pleasant are priceless. Team up with a friend who is also going through menopause, and you can give each other help and encouragement. You'll be surprised how much of a buzz it will give you. It can also help to know that you're not alone and that other women are going through menopause too and feel just like you. That's the beauty of joining my virtual Six-Week Natural Menopause program: women come together as a supportive community, and it makes the journey much more fun.

Be Future Positive

Being optimistic about the future is more likely to bring positive results than thinking about how good things used to be. There is lots of evidence to show that those who see life as a glass half full, rather than half empty, stand a much better chance of feeling content and fulfilled as they go into midlife. So, if your thoughts are veering toward the negative, indulge in some positive thinking when you wake up and before you go to sleep at night. Form a vivid picture of your happy, attractive self, going through the rest of life being incredibly positive, and start looking at things through these positive eyes. You'll feel so much better about life!

Spend time imagining yourself in great physical and mental shape, looking and feeling great with good things happening to you. If you have children who have now left home, you might imagine re-creating the romance of those first heady days you spent with your partner, enjoying the company of new friends, or even starting a new relationship. Perhaps your daydreams will center on success at work, going back to work, starting a new hobby, or fulfilling a lifetime ambition.

Whatever you focus on, make the images in your mind so realistic that you actually start to feel you are experiencing the situation. If you find this hard to do, try clipping pictures from magazines, or make a Pinterest board or a collage of some of your favorite photos. It may take some practice, but once you get the hang of it, it will become like watching a movie. Remember that if you feel positive about yourself, people are much more likely to react positively toward you.

Live Your Dream

Realizing your dreams requires an effort. Some people say there's no point in dreaming because you can't control your destiny. But evidence shows that positive thinking and visualization can go a long way toward getting you where you would like to be.

Take five or ten minutes each day to focus on your goals. The best time for this is first thing in the morning and last thing at night, so start and finish your day visualizing yourself just the way you would like to be — happy, fulfilled, looking forward to good things in the future, or whatever takes your fancy. Visualization is an acquired skill, so if it doesn't immediately happen in Technicolor and your mind keeps wandering, stick with it; eventually you'll get it. You have nothing to lose, and it's a positive way to begin and end each day.

This is a fun activity that allows you to portray your life the way you want it and design your dreams. It beats sitting around waiting for things to happen to you or just accepting what comes your way. There is a great deal of good living to be enjoyed in this new and exciting phase of your life, but you have to recognize that you are the architect of your life, not a victim of circumstances.

Lorraine's Story

Lorraine is a midwife who felt like she had reached the end of the road when menopause hit. I had helped her overcome PMS symptoms years ago, so she decided to ask for my help with her menopause.

Many of my relatives died young, so I had the sense that I needed to live life to the full, but I felt too bad to live the dream. I felt suicidal when I was going through my menopause. I felt worthless, and I had very frightening panic attacks.

I am a trained midwife and qualified complementary medicine practitioner and had really been enjoying my work until I started feeling unwell. I was finding it very difficult to work, as I wasn't able to focus or concentrate, which made me feel like I was compromising other people's lives.

When I think about it now, I hadn't felt well for years and suffered from a lack of sunshine in the winter. I had started getting hot flashes and night sweats even though I was only in my mid-forties, and I was so tired in the mornings that I struggled to get out of bed. I was feeling depressed, which was uncharacteristic for me, and had been put on antidepressants. During the day I ate tons of chocolate and junk food, and I blotted out my evenings by drinking as much as a bottle of wine. My libido had vanished, maybe because sex had become painful as my vagina was so dry. I had put on masses of weight, felt constantly bloated and anxious, and often had palpitations that made me feel dizzy. It felt like my whole body ached, and I longed to feel normal.

I had blood tests and was given HRT by my doctor, but it didn't suit me, so I came off it. I found I only had one week a month when I felt normal. My stress levels would increase, coupled with anxiety and forgetfulness, and my tolerance decreased. I eventually got signed off work as I was simply unable to function; in fact I had a complete breakdown.

One day, while I was lying in bed wondering how I was going to get through the day, I remembered that Maryon Stewart had helped me over my PMS symptoms in the nineties and again after my hysterectomy at age thirty, so I wondered if she would be able to help me reclaim my health again at midlife. I got in touch and signed up for a new program. She designed a program for me to follow. We didn't just talk about my diet, my excessive consumption of alcohol, or my lack of exercise, but we delved deeply into my life and what I really wanted out of my life. I remember telling Maryon that I dreamed of moving to live in a warmer climate.

I followed Maryon's recommendations as closely as I could. I started exercising again, although it took a while to get back to running, as I felt too tired. At Maryon's suggestion I made a vision board with my husband and filled it with pictures of life in Malta, and I made a gratitude list. Within four weeks I had lost seven pounds in weight, the hot flashes had stopped, my bowels had improved, my energy was returning, and we had booked a trip to Malta.

Within a matter of a weeks I felt much more like myself. I took some time out to look after myself and investigate the possibility of moving to Malta. My energy returned, I got back to running regularly, and my libido returned. That was a year ago. I'm happy to report that we now live in Malta and once again have a fully functioning personal relationship. I have a new job as a midwife, my menopause symptoms have gone, and for the first time in my life I feel at peace. I am once again so grateful to Maryon for her wise advice.

Reaching Your Goals

By the end of week 6, your routine should be established. You should also be experiencing relief from many of your symptoms, particularly hot flashes and night sweats. You should be feeling more energetic as a result of improved sleep and a healthier diet, including fewer stimulants.

It's important, though, to remember that my Six-Week Natural Menopause Solution was created from my tried and tested five-month program. After following the program for six weeks, women usually report feeling significantly better, seeing a light at the end of the tunnel. But it's very important to continue following the recommendations for several months to get the full benefit of the "midlife refuel." Even if you feel symptom-free within six weeks, I urge you to continue on your recovery journey for at least five months.

Part II

A NEW
BEGINNING

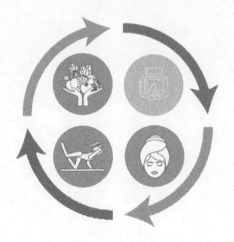

The chapters in this part of the book are not keyed to specific weeks in the Six-Week Natural Menopause Solution. Instead, each one takes an in-depth look at specific aspects of physical and mental well-being during menopause, and how to continue feeling great in midlife and beyond.

Chapter 7

MENOPAUSE IN THE WORKPLACE

Turning fifty should be cause for celebration. Many women will have successfully navigated the major challenges in life, such as establishing a career and raising a family. They are at the peak of their powers, likely earning more than ever before, and they should feel confident about coping with life. Instead, we are seeing lost workdays, a hit on the economy, and relationships under strain. A whole cohort of women is living in misery due to menopause.

According to the American Congress of Obstetricians and Gynecologists, an estimated 6,000 US women reach menopause every day. In all, 27 million women in the United States — 20 percent of the workforce — are experiencing menopause each year. *Forbes* magazine predicts that in 2025, over 1 billion women will be experiencing menopause around the world. That's 12 percent of the entire world population! At least 75 percent of them will experience hot flashes and night sweats, and among women experiencing menopause symptoms, the loss of productivity at work will be nearly 60 percent greater than among women not experiencing symptoms. The cost of this lost productivity and the burden on healthcare systems is estimated at more than $810 billion.

Menopause has traditionally been associated with the classic discomforts of night sweats, sleep deprivation, and muddled thinking. But it has deeper repercussions for both our personal and professional lives. In a survey of over one thousand working women that my team and I undertook in 2017, 80 percent reported suffering moderate to severe menopausal symptoms. Fifty percent of respondents said menopause had caused stress and strain on their close relationships; 60 percent reported lower self-esteem and a dip in confidence.

The survey found that despite women having more freedom and disposable income at midlife than previous generations, lack of knowledge about and effective treatment for menopause was draining them of money, happiness, and productivity. Eighty-four percent of respondents said their productivity at work was reduced; 75 percent felt their productivity was reduced for more than a week every month. This equates to 280 million less-productive workdays per year in the UK alone. Surprisingly, only 20 percent of the respondents took any time off work to deal with the symptoms.

Our workplace survey coincided with a government study released the same week, titled *The Effects of Menopause Transition on Women's Economic Participation in the UK*. The authors analyzed 104 international publications published from 1990 to March 2016 on the effects of menopause symptoms on women, the workplace, and the economy. I reviewed their study for the *Daily Mail* and concluded that the report contained a great deal of information about the problem and not much about the solution. The authors agreed. (One of the authors is Professor Jo Brewis, whose story appears on page 141.)

In a UK Trades Union Congress (TUC) study published in 2018, 78 percent of women surveyed said they avoided disclosing menopause symptoms to their line managers. When asked the reasons, 67 percent expressed concern that managers would link their situation to their performance at work, and 35 percent cited embarrassment. The authors of the TUC study argue that there is a robust business case for employer intervention to support women in menopause, as few companies offer any such support.

> I am now probably my most creative in years and can write with ease and actually enjoy my work.
>
> — Barbara Gustafson

Many women leave the workplace because of menopause symptoms, and a much greater number consider doing so at some point. The cost in lost productivity and talent is massive but has so far gone unaccounted for. The stresses associated with trying to continue performing at a high level when feeling subpar compound the physical, cognitive, and emotional symptoms of menopause.

In addition, some women experience discrimination as a result of their symptoms. There have been a few successful cases in the UK where women have taken their employers to court for discrimination over their menopause. One woman was dismissed for poor performance due to lack of concentration; when she sued, alleging discrimination, the court ruled in her favor, agreeing that it was unlikely that a man would be dismissed under similar circumstances. Although there have not yet been any similar cases in the US, it won't be too long before this trend crosses the Pond.

I'm all in favor of this, as it lifts the taboo on menopause, giving women permission to own up to being menopausal and get support. The next step is to provide constructive help to women in the workplace, so that instead of being dismissed as erratic and whiny during menopause, they are provided with science-based tools to overcome their symptoms. With this in mind my team and I have already started working with companies, including CISCO, Bank of America, and Virgin Healthcare, to offer workplace programs that help women to understand what's going on in their bodies and how to overcome symptoms.

The program also focuses on helping men, as colleagues and managers, better understand what happens at menopause so they can be supportive. Our surveys show that women shy away from opening up about menopause in the workplace, so we are encouraging them to follow a strategy to increase understanding and get support.

Jo's Story

Professor Jo Brewis, one of the coauthors of the UK government report on menopause in the workplace in the UK, was feeling scared about her ability to perform at work when we met because of cognitive difficulties associated with menopause.

I am a coauthor of a twenty-six-year review of menopause in the workplace. I met Maryon Stewart at a conference on menopause. At the time I was secretly scared stiff that I had early-onset Alzheimer's, as I had an inability to remember anything. I also felt confused, was constipated, and, for the first time in my life, had spots all over my chin, which made me very self-conscious.

I enrolled in Maryon's Six-Week Natural Menopause Solution, as I was desperate to overcome my brain fog and other symptoms. As an academic I need to be able to remember things and concentrate on whatever I am doing. My job is also very varied, so I constantly move between tasks in a day. Not being able to recall people's names or focus on a paper I was writing or a lecture I was preparing was proving to be incredibly difficult.

It took three weeks for me to begin to feel better following a natural program. My digestion is so much better, and my constipation vanished. And my state of mind is so much better too. My memory has returned. I focus better, and my skin has cleared, so I'm once again spot-free. I am also generally calmer, so if I've been concentrating hard for many hours and I do fog up, I have learned to give myself a break. If I relax, then whatever I am trying to remember usually comes to me, or my focus returns. Following Maryon's program, I know I look better, as people are forever commenting on it. I feel more confident, almost a new woman, and I've now been made head of department at my university, which would have been unthinkable not long before

As a coauthor of the government report "The Effects of Menopause Transition on Women's Economic Participation in the UK," I am aware that most emphasis is placed on the problem rather than the solution. So often women are left with inadequate help or advice. They don't seem to be supported at home: my own partner used to make fun of my memory loss. Some more-forward-thinking companies are introducing policies and being more supportive of women going through menopause, but much more focus needs to be placed on the solution rather than just labeling women as menopausal.

Talking to Your Boss

One of our recent surveys shows that 45 percent of women find it hard to talk about menopause with their boss as well as their colleagues; 54 percent of respondents felt that doing so would make them look less capable in the workplace, and 45 percent didn't feel their boss would understand. In another survey carried out by the British TV broadcaster ITV with the charity Wellbeing of Women, 25 percent of women said they had thought about leaving their jobs due to menopausal symptoms.

The time has clearly come to raise employer awareness and establish better workplace support systems, but meanwhile the first step is for women to start the conversation themselves.

You may feel awkward, embarrassed, and anxious you won't be taken seriously. It's often hard enough talking about symptoms to your doctor, friends, and family, let alone your line manager, especially if it's a man. But remember, your manager and colleagues want you to be at your best at work, so take a deep breath and get talking. Menopause is a natural transition in life, and you deserve to be listened to. Here's how to plan for and start the conversation.

Document your situation: Keep a diary of your menopause symptoms, how they're affecting you at work, and what you're doing to manage them.

Focus on solutions: How would you like your line manager to support you? Think about any practical and reasonable adjustments that would help. Could you work from home or come in to work later some days if poor sleep is an issue? If the temperature in your office is making hot flashes worse, could you have a fan or move to a desk near an air-conditioning unit or a window you can open?

Check out available support: Does your employer have a menopause policy? If not, what support is already available? Look at existing policies on sick leave, disability, and flexible working policies. Your employer may also offer an employee assistance program, which can provide access to counseling services to help with symptoms like anxiety and low mood.

Schedule a meeting: This means you'll have the time to talk, ideally in a private place.

Prepare: This is probably not going to be the easiest workplace conversation you have had, so it's important to plan it. You could even role-play with a trusted friend. Going for a walk before the meeting may help you relax. Think about how you are going to approach the subject.

Describe the problem: In the meeting, explain carefully how your symptoms are affecting you. You might mention that disturbed sleep is making it hard for you to think clearly; that fear of an embarrassing hot flash makes you anxious during meetings; or that you're experiencing a lack of focus and concentration that makes it harder for you to take decisions.

Offer solutions: Explain that this is a transition for you, and describe constructive steps you're taking to overcome your symptoms. You might say you are learning how to have a "midlife refuel" so that you can get turbocharged for the future. A little humor might help. Have some solutions to offer, such as asking for more flexible working hours for the next month to give yourself a chance to recover. If hot flashes are a problem, you could suggest working from home, where you can regulate the temperature of your workspace without having to ask for a cooler environment at work.

Follow up: At the end of the meeting put a time in the diary to meet again, whether that's to agree a way forward, monitor progress, or give an update.

Be patient: Don't expect an immediate answer. Your boss may not be well in-formed about menopause or how best to support you. Allow them time to digest what you've talked about and possibly seek advice from your employer's human resources or occupational health staff.

Be professional: Above all, remember this is just two professional people hav-ing a conversation. It's in both your best interests to find a good solution.

Talking to Your Colleagues

Some women are happy to talk to colleagues about their menopause, others aren't. It's your choice. But it can help to open up and talk about it. Your colleagues, especially if they are male or younger than you, may not know much about midlife changes. Explaining your symptoms and their effect on your mental and physical well-being will help them understand this important transition in your life and make them better equipped to sup-port you.

Choose a time: You may prefer to have a one-to-one conversation or talk to a couple of colleagues at a time. Do whatever feels the most comfortable for you.

Be honest: Colleagues may have noticed that you are not your usual self, so explain how you are feeling and how it is affecting your work and moods.

Explain your symptoms: Colleagues may not know much about symptoms of menopause, so explain the causes and the triggers, and talk frankly. They may be able to help. For example, if you find your work environment too hot, one of your colleagues may be sitting in a cooler area and be happy to swap.

Put them at their ease: Encourage them to ask questions about menopause. Once they have the answers, they may be more understanding and supportive.

Show appreciation: Thank them for their time and support. And let them know that if they want to talk more you are always open to the conversation.

Managing Menopause Symptoms at Work

- Give yourself plenty of time. Rushing because you are late or short of time is likely to bring on hot flashes.

- Stay hydrated. Have cool water on hand, and drink some as soon as you feel a hot flash coming on. Consider using an insulated cup to keep the water cool.
- Keep wet wipes in your bag and desk drawer, and have a portable fan available to help cool yourself down.
- Layer your clothing so you can peel off as needed while still looking professional.
- Keep calm. If you feel stressed, focus on breathing slowly and taking a moment to regroup.
- Avoid caffeinated drinks, and let hot drinks cool before drinking them, so that you minimize hot flashes. See page 168 for suggested alternatives.
- Stay nourished. Consume wholesome, phyto-rich food and snacks at regular intervals.
- Communicate with your managers and colleagues about what you're experiencing. That way you get increased support and understanding while you recover.
- Do at least one session of formal relaxation each day (see page 90) to help reduce work stress.

> Before Maryon's program I was contemplating leaving the workplace due to my brain fog and confusion. Now I'm over that and I've been made head of department at my university.
>
> — Professor Jo Brewis

Chapter 8

COMPLEMENTARY THERAPIES

Although it might seem like the cards are stacked against you, following my Six-Week Natural Menopause Solution will have taught you how to get your brain chemistry and hormones back into balance. But if you feel in need of some extra help to deal with specific symptoms, you may want to consider complementary alternative therapies. I often refer clients to other practitioners for treatment. For example, acupuncture works wonders for speeding up healing; cranial-sacral therapy, and cranial osteopathy in the UK, can be a godsend if you have problems with your back; and neck massage is a wonderful muscle soother that can help to accelerate recovery.

Acupuncture and Acupressure

Many problems related to menopause may respond to acupuncture. This treatment is based on the idea that the body has channels of energy that can become blocked, leading to symptoms ranging from irritability and anxiety to insomnia and headaches. An acupuncturist uses fine needles inserted at specific points on your body, known as meridians, to help unblock these energy channels. Acupressure, which involves applying pressure at certain points on your body with the fingertips, can also be a useful tool, and it's one you can use at home. Nine percent of the participants in my midlife survey tried a course of acupuncture, and 74 percent of these found it helpful.

Aromatherapy Massage

While I don't buy into the idea that aromatherapy, or even a combination of aromatherapy and massage, can cure everything from acne to ingrown toenails, some research suggests that it might be a useful tool during menopause. Aromatherapy involves the application of essential oils, which are either massaged into the skin or inhaled. These oils are thought to stimulate the olfactory system in the brain, which then sends messages to the part of the brain that controls our emotions, which in turn causes neurotransmitters to be released into the body that make us feel calmer and more relaxed. Apart from the potentially therapeutic effect of aromatherapy, just taking time out for yourself to go for a massage can be good for you.

Emotional Freedom Techniques

Emotional freedom techniques (EFT), or tapping, as the practice is often called, is an alternative treatment for physical pain in conjunction with underlying emotional issues, including anxiety, that has shown good results in clinical trials. It's often referred to as psychological acupressure.

EFT combines cognitive behavioral therapy, focusing on a specific symptom or fear, with manual stimulation on acupressure points, tapping with your fingertips at specific points on your face and body to clear persistent symptoms or counterproductive thoughts or feelings, including depression, anxiety, panic attacks, joint pain, and digestive problems. It's easy to practice at home. There are many good books on the subject as well as short instructional videos on YouTube. There are also many registered practitioners. It's a useful technique to have at your disposal even if you are just trying to relieve a headache.

Herbal Medicine

Various forms of herbal medicine have been used for thousands of years to help treat all kinds of ailments. Many herbs have now undergone clinical trials to examine how they work and why, and I have incorporated more herbal medicine into my program. The herbs found to be most effective in combating symptoms of menopause are maca root, red clover, black cohosh, ginseng, St. John's wort, sage, dong quai, valerian, and vitex (see chapter 4). Of the 24 percent of the participants in our midlife survey who had tried herbs, 80 percent found them useful.

Homeopathy

While conventional medicine aims to treat people with a drug that counteracts the effects of a condition or disease, homoeopathy aims to treat like with like by administering a minuscule quantity of a substance thought to provoke the symptoms. The word *homeopathy* comes from the Greek words for *similar* and *disease*. This treatment is said to stimulate the body to fight back against the symptoms.

Sepia and sulfur are two of the many homeopathic remedies that may be recommended for hot flashes and night sweats. There is also a wide choice of remedies for poor memory, depression, insomnia, anxiety attacks, irritability, headaches, and confusion. Fourteen percent of the women in our midlife survey had tried homoeopathy, of whom 76 percent found it helpful.

Cranial-Sacral Therapy

Cranial-sacral (or craniosacral) therapy and cranial osteopathy involve gentle manipulation of the body's soft tissues. They can also help with chronic back, head, and neck pain and have been shown to reduce hot flashes. Treatment for women suffering menopausal symptoms is often aimed at improving function of the pituitary gland at the base of the brain, which controls the adrenal glands and consequently affects many of the body's functions.

Cautions

When opting for any complementary therapy, it is important to find an experienced and qualified practitioner. These days, the more widely recognized complementary specialties have official associations that keep registers of qualified practitioners. You can contact these groups and read about registered practitioners online to see whether they would be a good fit for you, or ask for a recommendation in your local health store.

What the Research Says

Years ago when I first did a literature search, there were only a few small studies to support some complementary therapies, but the evidence base now contains many encouraging studies that document the effectiveness of various therapies in relieving menopause symptoms.

There are several reports of the successful treatment of menopause symptoms with acupuncture and traditional Chinese medicine (TCM), which uses herbal remedies extensively. One review showed that acupuncture can reduce menopause-related sleep disturbances. Another study reviewed controlled clinical trials of TCM for hot flashes occurring in conjunction with sleep, cognitive function, mood, or pain. The study concluded that TCM showed promising results for treating mood and pain symptoms co-occurring with hot flashes.

A comparison of acupuncture with sham acupuncture, traditional Chinese medicine, and a placebo showed that acupuncture is effective in reducing both the frequency and severity of hot flashes. The Chinese herbal medicine, however, was not effective.

A study from Iran shows that acupressure can be used as a complementary treatment to relieve sleep disorders in menopausal women.

Another study has shown that acupuncture, used in an integrated system that includes therapeutic techniques such as diet therapy and self-massage, can reduce hot flashes and sleep disturbances in postmenopausal women.

Also of interest is a multinational review of homeopathic medicines prescribed for menopausal symptoms. Remedies including *Lachesis mutus*, belladonna, *Sepia officinalis*, sulfur, and *Sanguinaria canadensis* were the most frequently prescribed. This observational study revealed a significant reduction in the frequency of hot flashes and the daily discomfort they caused. Ninety percent of the women who took homeopathic remedies reported the disappearance or lessening of their symptoms, most within fifteen days of starting homeopathic treatment.

Finally, there is evidence that aromatherapy massage can also help menopausal symptoms. A study involving ninety women compared the effects of massage, aromatherapy massage, and no treatment. Psychological symptoms were assessed before and after intervention. Both aromatherapy massage and massage were shown to reduce psychological symptoms, but aromatherapy massage was more effective than regular massage. Another study found aromatherapy massage more effective than regular massage for other menopausal symptoms as well.

Chapter 9

LOOKING AFTER
YOUR HEART

B efore menopause, women's risk of heart disease is significantly lower than that of men of the same age. Researchers are not sure why, but it's thought that estrogen may have a protective effect.

After menopause, women's risk of heart disease — including atherosclerosis (furring and hardening of the arteries), high blood pressure, angina, heart attack, and stroke — is similar to that of men, and around 30 percent will develop heart disease. It seems that menopause brings changes in the level of fats in the blood known as lipids, which determine cholesterol level. There are two components of cholesterol: high density lipoproteins (HDL), which are associated with a beneficial, cleansing effect in the bloodstream, and low-density lipoproteins (LDL), which encourage fat and mineral deposits, known as plaque, to accumulate on the walls of arteries, causing them to narrow and clog up.

In postmenopausal women, as a direct result of estrogen deficiency, LDL cholesterol appears to increase, while HDL decreases. Elevated LDL and total cholesterol levels are linked to a higher risk of stroke, heart attack, and death. Fortunately, there are easy and effective measures we can take to protect our heart health.

Quiz: What's Your Risk of Heart Disease?

- Do you smoke?
- Do you exercise less than three or four times a week?

- Do you eat a lot of fatty foods, such as fried foods, including French fries, cheese, hamburgers, and ice cream?
- Do you consume more than two servings of red meat each week?
- Are you overweight?
- Do you have high blood pressure?
- Is your cholesterol count high?
- Do you drink more than one five-ounce glass of wine per day (or the equivalent in other alcoholic drinks)?
- Do you eat oily fish less than twice a week?
- Do you eat fewer than five portions of fruit and vegetables a day?

If you answered yes to more than three questions, follow the guidelines in this chapter to switch to a heart-friendly lifestyle. Don't forget to make a note of your score in your Natural Menopause Solution worksheet.

Action Plan
Follow a Healthy-Heart Diet

We have known for years that meat and dairy products contain saturated fats (hard fats) that can contribute to atherosclerosis, so these foods should be eaten in moderation. Also harmful are trans fats, many of which are chemically altered types of fat created from polyunsaturated fats such as sunflower oil. Trans fats, used as ingredients in processed foods such as burgers, sausages, pies, cakes, and cookies, were banned from food production in the US and Canada in 2018 but are still permitted in some other countries, including the UK and Australia.

According to research as far back as 1990, diet can be as effective in combating atherosclerosis as drugs or surgery. In the study, a group of people with severely blocked arteries went on a very low-fat vegetarian diet along with an exercise and meditation program, at the end of which the plaque in their arteries was found to be reduced.

Research suggests that isoflavones can reduce the risk of coronary heart disease. A meta-analysis of the effects of soy protein containing isoflavones on blood lipids showed beneficial reductions in serum total cholesterol, LDL cholesterol, and triglycerides, with increases in beneficial HDL cholesterol.

Not all fats are harmful. Monounsaturated fats, found in olive oil, and the omega-3 essential fatty acids (found in flaxseeds, pumpkin, and walnuts as alpha-linolenic acid, or ALA) need to be included in the diet. The body converts ALA to eicosapentaenoic acid (EPA) and docosahexaenoic acid (DHA), found naturally in oily fish, to produce anti-inflammatory prostaglandins. Most experts now agree that to reduce your risk of heart disease, you need to limit your intake of saturated animal fats, increase your intake of omega-3 EFAs, and include heart-healthy monounsaturated fats, such as those found in virgin olive oil, in your diet. You should also try to eat oily fish, such as salmon, mackerel, herring, sardines, and anchovies at least twice a week. The omega-3 EFAs in these fish can help protect against heart and circulatory disease.

Coconut oil has recently been widely promoted as a healthy alternative to other cooking fats. While there is little robust research to justify some of the health claims made about it, it is true that coconut oil is a medium-chain triglyceride (MCT), which means that it's used as an energy source, and therefore less is stored as fat. However, it also contains saturated fats, so moderation is needed. Coconut oil has a high melting point, meaning that it's safe and stable to use for high-temperature cooking, unlike sunflower or corn oils.

For heart health, it's important to drink alcohol only in moderation, as it can raise blood pressure and cholesterol levels. It's also important to eat at least five portions of fruit and vegetables every day. This ensures an adequate intake of dietary fiber, which helps eliminate the "bad" LDL cholesterol from the body. Fruits and vegetables are also loaded with antioxidants, which help protect the arteries from damage and keep blood flowing smoothly.

Cut Down on Salt

Table salt, or sodium chloride, is associated with fluid retention — you may have noticed puffiness and bloating following a very salty meal. Some of the fluid retained as a result of excessive sodium intake is pulled into our blood vessels, increasing the volume of fluid inside the vessels and causing high blood pressure (hypertension). Over time, high blood pressure overstretches and damages blood vessel walls and contributes to the buildup of harmful arterial plaque that impedes blood flow. High blood pressure increases the risk of heart failure, as it forces the heart to work harder to pump blood through the body. It can also lead to strokes. High blood pressure is known as the "silent killer" because it often has no apparent symptoms until a serious or fatal heart attack or stroke occurs. Ninety percent of American adults are expected to develop high blood pressure during their lifetime.

For many people, controlling salt intake is an effective means of managing blood pressure. Avoid eating salty processed foods or adding salt to food while cooking or at the table. Use other condiments, including herbs and mild spices, to add flavor. Seagreens is a great salt substitute derived from seaweed. It provides a number of good nutrients without the downside of sodium found in regular salt.

Get Moving

Regular aerobic exercise at least five days a week will help keep your heart and circulatory system in good shape. See chapter 4 for recommendations on starting an exercise program.

Give Up Smoking

If you are still puffing away, give up now, for the sake of your heart. Smoke-damaged arteries attract fatty deposits that restrict the blood flow to your heart. Smoking also damages the lungs, making it harder for the heart to supply the body with oxygen. In addition, it can make blood stickier and more likely to clot, which can lead to a blockage in an artery resulting in a heart attack or stroke.

Five "Hearty" Things to Do Today

1. Leave your car at home and walk to the supermarket or work.
2. Go for a thirty-minute walk at lunchtime.
3. Listen to some music and get dancing.
4. Use only a small amount of butter or a low-fat spread on your toast.
5. Don't put the salt on the table or add excessive amounts of salt to food when cooking.

What the Research Says

It was discovered almost by accident in the late 1960s that soy protein lowers cholesterol levels. Researchers who were looking at whether soy protein could be a palatable alternative to meat discovered a marked reduction in cholesterol levels in people who consumed a lot of soy.

Almost a decade later, researchers at the University of Milan discovered that consuming soy protein lowered cholesterol levels by an average of 14 percent within two weeks and 21 percent within three weeks. The Italians are so convinced about the value of soy in lowering cholesterol that soy protein and soy protein isolate are now provided free of charge by the Italian National Health Service to people with high cholesterol.

In 1999, the researcher Kenneth Carrol analyzed the results of forty published studies on the effects of soy on cholesterol. He found that thirty-four of the studies showed a drop in levels of LDL cholesterol of 15 percent or more.

Another study in the US by Kenneth Setchell confirmed that it is possible to raise HDL cholesterol and lower LDL cholesterol by following a soy-rich diet. The twelve-week study followed forty-three postmenopausal women who consumed a diet that included 60–70 mg of isoflavones each day. Isoflavones were found to provide the added benefit of preventing plaque buildup, reducing the possibility of an arterial blockage.

In October 1999, the US Food and Drug Administration (FDA) approved a health claim for soy protein and its role in reducing the risk of coronary heart disease. This same approval was eventually granted by the UK authorities. Labels on food products containing at least 6.25 mg of soy protein per serving may claim that the product may reduce the risk of heart disease when consumed in conjunction with a low-fat, low-cholesterol diet.

A multicenter study published in December 2005 suggests that soy-enriched foods may help protect women from heart disease after menopause by reducing inflammation. It is thought that before menopause, estrogen protects women from heart disease by lowering the amount of inflammatory substances in the blood. A group of 117 European women were given either isoflavone-enriched or normal cereal bars. The results of the study suggest that soy protects some women more than others, depending on their genetic makeup.

Researchers from the University of Guelph in Canada decided to examine the effects of a reduction in overall cholesterol on heart health in a group of postmenopausal women. The women received 2.8 grams of DHA a day for twenty-eight days. Their study, published in the *American Journal of Clinical Nutrition*, found that DHA supplementation was associated with a 20 percent reduction in serum triacylglycerol (unused stored fats), an 8 percent increase in HDLs ("good" cholesterol), a 28 percent lower overall ratio of serum triacylglycerol to HDLs, and a 7 percent decrease in resting heart rate.

Chapter 10

BUILDING NEW BONE

Many women assume that when their menopause symptoms stop, they are on safe ground. Sadly, without the protective effect of estrogen, we face some long-term risks to our health. As well as being at greater risk of heart disease, we start to lose more bone each year than we make, increasing our risk of the bone-thinning disease osteoporosis.

Osteoporosis involves a loss of calcium (the mineral in bones) and collagen (the gluey protein that helps strengthen them). As a result, the fine, honeycomb texture of normal, healthy bones is replaced by gaping holes. Bones lose their ability to absorb shock and may become so weak that even a small impact or fall can cause a fracture.

What causes osteoporosis? You may not think of bones as living tissue, but they go through a constant process of renewal. Until the age of about thirty-five, we generally make as much new bone as we lose, keeping the scales in balance. But from then on, we tend to lose around 1 percent of our total bone mass each year until we reach menopause. From that point, bone loss accelerates a further 2 to 3 percent per year for up to ten years.

This bone loss is partly due to falling levels of estrogen, as one of the key roles of this important hormone is to maintain bone mass. The rate of bone loss is estimated to be about 70 percent due to our genetic makeup. But lifestyle factors are also involved, some of which can be managed to help maintain the strength of our bones for life.

Factors That Build Strong Bones

- Diet, especially the intake of calcium during the growing years
- Physical activity, particularly weight-bearing exercise
- Hormonal factors, particularly estrogen balance
- Genetic factors, which determine the size of bones and muscles
- Optimal levels of nutrients, including calcium, magnesium, boron, vitamin K2, vitamin D, and omega-3 and omega-6 essential fatty acids

Action Plan
Assess Your Diet

Building bone is a complex biological process. Calcium is the main component, but magnesium, phosphorus, boron, and vitamins C, D, and K2 are also important. Magnesium helps the body to absorb and use calcium, and establishing a healthy balance of these two minerals is vital. Vitamin K2 is also necessary for calcium metabolism. It is produced in small quantities by gut bacteria in the large intestine; it is also found in fermented foods, including soy, and in animal products, including chicken and eggs.

Dairy products are rich sources of calcium, but they contain almost no magnesium. So how do cows grow such large, strong bones after weaning? They eat grass. And this is the key: any green, leafy vegetable, such as watercress, kale, broccoli, or cabbage, provides the perfect balance of calcium and magnesium. Nuts and seeds also provide balanced amounts of these two minerals. See page 82 for further details about nutritional supplements and recommended doses.

Get Phyto Rich

In addition to all their other health benefits, plant phytoestrogens have been shown to increase the number of new bone cells made after menopause. Good sources include soybeans (especially edamame beans), tofu, soy milk, flaxseeds, and to a lesser degree lentils, chickpeas, and mung beans.

Eat Prunes

Consuming five prunes a day (50 g) for six months has been shown to reduce bone loss and lower risk of osteoporosis. To prevent gas and bloating, choose prunes that haven't been preserved with sulfur dioxide.

Be Sunny

Vitamin D helps your gut absorb the calcium you need for bone health, but it's one of the most common nutritional deficiencies among women. The action of sunlight on our skin provides the main source, so it's important to get a little sunshine regularly, without over-doing it. Those with fair skin should apply sunscreen after ten minutes of sun exposure, and those with medium or dark skin can be exposed for a little longer.

Sunlight alone is now not thought to be sufficient to keep our vitamin D levels in an optimum range. The US National Institutes of Health (NIH) recommends that women over fifty take a supplement containing 600 IU of vitamin D3 each day. However, in nutritional circles this is considered insufficient.

Quiz: How Strong Are Your Bones?

- In your childhood and teens, did you consume a diet low in calcium (and lacking dairy products)?
- Do you regularly consume red meat and dairy products rather than vegetarian sources of protein?
- Did you experience an early menopause, spontaneously or following surgery?
- Do you have a history of thyroid or other hormonal problems?
- Have you been underweight or suffered an eating disorder, such as anorexia or bulimia?
- Have you always had a petite build?
- Do you smoke ten or more cigarettes per day?
- Have there been times in your life when you regularly drank alcohol to excess (more than the equivalent of seven glasses of wine per week)?
- Do you only rarely perform weight-bearing exercise?

- Do you lead a sedentary lifestyle?
- Have you had periods of highly strenuous physical activity in your life, for instance, as an elite athlete or a ballet dancer?
- Have you ever taken steroid drugs for an extended period?
- Have you suffered more than one fracture since your menopause?
- Has a close relative suffered from osteoporosis?
- Have you experienced a chronic illness that affected your digestion, kidney, or liver function?
- Did you ever stop having periods, especially when you were young?

If you answered yes to just one of these questions, you may be at risk of osteoporosis. If you answered yes to more than two questions, you need to start making changes to your diet and lifestyle as soon as you can. Don't forget to enter your score in your Natural Menopause Solution worksheet.

Go for Essential Fatty Acids

Research suggests that foods rich in omega-3 and omega-6 essential fatty acids may help us absorb calcium from food. Omega-3s are found in fish oils, oily fish (salmon, mackerel, herring, sardines, anchovies, chia seeds, and some oils, such as soy and walnut oil). Good sources of omega-6 EFAs include walnut, olive, and coconut oil, almonds, green leafy vegetables, flaxseeds, and whole grains.

Foods to Avoid

Try not to include too much animal protein, salt, or caffeine in your diet, as excessive quantities can reduce your body's ability to absorb and retain calcium. Excessive alcohol is also thought to interfere with calcium metabolism and affect bone-building cells, resulting in loss of bone density.

Exercise Regularly

Exercise plays a vital part in keeping bones healthy. Try to include both aerobic activity and strengthening exercises in your regular routine. Weight-bearing activities that cause a slight impact on the bones are more effective in maintaining bone health than activities where your body weight is supported, such as swimming or cycling. Running, jogging, brisk walking, tennis, table tennis, jumping rope, and lifting weights are all good choices. Gentler alternatives include golf, gardening, and dancing. Aim for at least thirty to forty-five minutes of moderate exercise at least five times a week.

Strengthening exercises make it possible for you to target body parts such as the upper spine, hips, wrists, and ankles, which are more vulnerable to fractures. You can do these in a gym with weight-training equipment or at home with free weights. Pilates and yoga are also good for building strength, flexibility, and balance, lessening our chances of falling and fracturing bones as we age.

Your bone health can be checked with a bone density scan. Over the years my team and I have regularly seen good production of new bone in clients not taking hormone replacement therapy, but it does take several years to notice the difference on a bone density scan. Fifteen years ago, my own bone mass measured average for my age. That was quite a shock, as I expected it to be higher. Five years later, after doing regular weight-bearing exercise for over four years, I had another bone density scan and was delighted to find that my bone mass was now 17 percent above average for my age.

Findings of the Natural Health Advisory Service Osteoporosis Survey

At the Natural Health Advisory Service, my team and I carried out a survey of one thousand women to analyze the link between diet, lifestyle, and osteoporosis. The respondents varied in age from 18 to over 80; the average age was 55 years.

The survey revealed that many women are unaware of the nutritional and dietary requirements for preventing osteoporosis. Nearly 75 percent of the women were unaware that soy products should be incorporated into the diet to prevent osteoporosis. Over 50 percent were not fully aware of the importance of calcium in the form of dairy products, and 66 percent did not do enough exercise to maintain their bone health.

Joanne's Story

Joanne, a mother of two in her early forties from Toronto, Canada, was diagnosed with early-onset osteoporosis.

I went through an early menopause in my early forties. I had a bone density scan and was shocked to discover a 7 percent loss of bone mass in one year. I was advised to take long-term medication, but after reading one of Maryon Stewart's books, I decided to give myself a year of natural solutions before accepting the drugs as the solution.

I went and saw Maryon, who helped me refine my program. This involved making significant dietary changes, taking nutritional supplements, and doing daily weight-bearing exercises.

A year later, my follow-up bone density scan showed almost no further bone loss, and the advice this time was "Keep taking the tablets." I'm hoping that next year's scan will show I have made some new bone. I'm certainly feeling well and much fitter as a result of my new regimen.

What the Research Says

A recent review looked at studies on osteoporotic bone loss in relation to soy isoflavone intake from either diet or supplements, with an emphasis on the role of these compounds in the generation of new bone. It suggests that dietary soy isoflavones slow down menopause-induced bone loss and stimulate new bone formation.

Another study investigated the effectiveness of five different soy isoflavone supplements compared with risedronate, a bisphosphonate drug used in the treatment of osteoporosis, in preserving bone in a group of twenty-five women. Each participant took a supplement and risedronate for a fifty-day period, with a fifty-day washout period when changing supplements, and their bone calcium was measured after each cycle.

A daily supplement containing a total of 105 mg of isoflavones, in the forms of genistein, daidzein, and glycitein in the same proportions found in nature, was the most effective of the soy isoflavone supplements tested. This supplement increased bone retention by 7.6 percent. A dose of 53 mg of genistein daily increased bone retention by 3.4 percent. Although the isoflavone supplements were not as effective as risedronate, which increased bone retention by 15 percent, the results were encouraging, particularly because the supplements do not have the potential side effects of risedronate, which include gastric upset and hot flashes.

The researchers concluded that soy isoflavones, in the right dose and composition, are effective in promoting the growth of new bone in menopausal women. Compared with bisphosphonates and HRT, the use of soy isoflavones presents a minimal to negligible risk to menopausal women and can be used over the long term for some protection against bone loss.

A relatively recent study looked at the effects of AlgaeCal, a vitamin- and mineral-enhanced, plant-based, highly bioavailable form of calcium, in people who had purchased and used the supplement for one to seven years. AlgaeCal was linked to an annual increase of 1 percent in bone mineral density — a cumulative increase of 7.3 percent over seven years. Data from other sources, covering 16,289 women, suggested that the expected change in bone density in this group if they were not taking the supplement would be a loss of 0.4 percent of bone mass per year. The findings are consistent with previous short-term studies of this supplement. They suggest that taking AlgaeCal can lead to significant increases in total bone mineral density, whereas conventional calcium supplements may only slow down age-related decline.

The positive findings here on the safety and efficacy of AlgaeCal contrast with the reported adverse effects and decline in efficacy for bisphosphonates. There is some evidence, for instance, that use of bisphosphonates over three to five years is associated with fractures of the femur (the thighbone).

Researchers from the Harvard Medical School and the University of Connecticut collaborated on a study that compared the effects of AlgaeCal with the two best-known types of calcium supplements, calcium carbonate and calcium citrate. Compared to the other forms of calcium, AlgaeCal almost doubled the ability of the osteoblasts (the cells that build bone tissue) to produce new bone.

Strontium is a mineral similar to calcium, naturally present in trace amounts in the body (around 100 mcg in every gram of bone). It has been known since the 1950s to have a positive bone-building effect. In clinical trials on menopausal women with osteopenia, the precursor to osteoporosis, the product Strontium Boost, when used in addition to AlgaeCal, improved bone density a further 4 percent.

A study published in 2017 examining the role of exercise and sports in the prevention of osteoporosis demonstrated that walking, aerobic weight-bearing exercise, muscle-strengthening exercise, and weight-bearing plus muscle-strengthening exercises maintained or increased bone mineral density in postmenopausal women.

There is evidence that foods containing nutrients like vitamin K, boron, manganese, copper, and potassium can help to reduce bone loss. Fifty grams of dried prunes per day, for example, have been shown to reduce bone loss after six months.

Part III

LET'S EAT

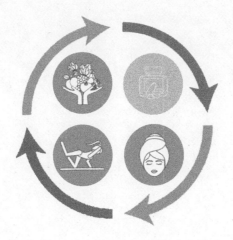

In this part of the book you will find dietary tools for creating your own Natural Menopause Solution. To help you follow a healthy eating plan, this part of the book includes sample menu plans; a collection of healthy, phyto-rich recipes; a list of selected ready-made phyto-rich and gluten-free foods and drinks; and a list of foods ranked according to their content of specific nutrients, to help you select foods that boost the nutrients you might be short of.

Chapter 11

PHYTO-RICH
MEAL PLANS

Plants such as soy, flaxseeds, and red clover are collectively known as phytoestrogen rich because they contain naturally occurring estrogens (isoflavones and lignans) that have been found to significantly reduce menopausal symptoms for many women.

You don't need to radically change your diet to increase your intake of these compounds — just make a few modifications. Look at the table "Isoflavone Content of Foods" in chapter 3 to identify phyto-rich foods that you enjoy eating, and then consider how you can easily include these in your diet. Many phyto-rich ingredients and convenience foods are readily available in supermarkets.

The suggested meal plans below are designed to help you incorporate more isoflavones and lignans into your daily menu. Following the meal plans are a number of simple but delicious recipes for you to try, all of which contain naturally occurring estrogen.

Diet Dos and Don'ts

Your goal is to restore estrogen levels and put back some of the nutrients that time and nature have depleted, including magnesium, zinc, B vitamins, Vitamin D, calcium, and essential fatty acids (EFAs).

Do

1. Include at least 100 mg of phytoestrogens in your daily diet. Their effects last only a few hours, so you should spread your intake throughout the day. The best sources are soy products and golden flaxseeds. Other sources, not as rich, include chickpeas, lentils, mung beans, alfalfa, sunflower seeds, pumpkin seeds, sesame seeds, rhubarb, and green and yellow vegetables. Adding two tablespoons of golden roasted flaxseeds to breakfast cereal, yogurt, or fruit salad is an easy way to get a "phyto fix." Flaxseeds are one of the richest sources of natural phytoestrogens and are also a good source of fiber, which can help alleviate constipation.

2. Eat at least five servings of fresh fruit and vegetables per day. These foods provide plenty of potassium and magnesium, plus small amounts of phytoestrogens. Where possible, buy organic products, or grow your own, to help ensure that your diet is as nutrient dense as possible.

3. Go for foods rich in calcium and magnesium, such as milk, green leafy vegetables, unsalted nuts and seeds, whole grains, and fish, including sardines and tuna.

4. Eat regularly. Three meals a day, with snacks as needed, help to ensure a balanced diet, as well as a steady flow of energy throughout the day.

5. Include approximately 50 grams of protein from animal or vegetarian sources in at least one meal a day. As low-protein diets jeopardize the balance of many nutrients, including calcium, B vitamins, and iron, I tend to recommend extra protein, especially for those who are exercising regularly.

6. Limit your consumption of red meat to one or two portions a week. Women tend not to digest meat so well at midlife, and reducing consumption of animal fats helps protect the heart and blood vessels. Go for fish, poultry, peas, beans, soy, and nuts instead.

7. Have a serving of dairy products each day to boost your intake of protein and calcium. You can add milk to your cereal or drinks, or eat cheese or yogurt. These foods provide calcium and protein. If you don't tolerate dairy products well, try another form of milk, such as soy, nut, or rice milk. Go for low-fat options if you need to lose weight.

8. Drink plenty of liquids, preferably the equivalent of at least eight glasses of water daily, which can include herbal and fruit teas. Rooibos tea, which can

also be prepared with milk to make chai, makes a good alternative to caffeinated black tea. Remember that very hot drinks may bring on a hot flash.

9. Consume two portions of oily fish per week, including salmon, mackerel, herring, and sardines, which are rich sources of omega-3 EFAs and help maintain hormone health as well as joint health.

10. Keep a supply of nutritious snacks to eat between meals if you get hungry. Phyto fix bars (see recipes), unsalted nuts and seeds, fresh fruit, and dried fruit are ideal. (Choose unsulfured dried fruit to prevent gas or bloating.)

12. Consider taking some of the nutritional supplements recommended in chapter 4 to help boost your nutrient levels in the short-term.

Don't

1. Don't go overboard on alcohol. Limit yourself to three drinks per week. Alcohol aggravates hot flashes and insomnia, and when consumed in excess can aggravate nutritional deficiencies.

2. Don't drink endless cups of coffee or black tea. Caffeine can aggravate hot flashes, as well as anxiety and insomnia. Even drinks labeled as decaffeinated usually contain a small amount of caffeine. Go for herbal alternatives instead.

3. Don't consume hot curry or other heavily spiced foods, as the spices, like hot drinks and alcohol, can bring on hot flashes.

4. Don't eat sugar or sweet junk foods, including sugar added to tea and coffee. Avoid candy, cakes, cookies, chocolate, jams, honey, ice cream, and soft drinks. Consumption of these foods and drinks may reduce the uptake of essential nutrients and cause water retention and bloating. Carbonated soft drinks containing phosphates may also impede the absorption of calcium.

5. Don't add salt while cooking or at the table. Our food already contains far more salt than we need. Excessive salt causes fluid retention and calcium loss from the body through the urine. Avoid highly salted foods like smoked fish and bacon. Use potassium-rich salt substitutes or other flavorings such as garlic, onion, kelp powder, fresh herbs, sesame powder, or other mild spices.

6. Don't eat foods containing wheat (including wheat bran), in the short term, if you feel bloated or experience gas or constipation.

7. Don't eat lots of fatty foods. Aim to get no more than 30 percent of your daily calories from fat. For most of us, this means reducing fat consumption by at

least 25 percent and reading product labels to look for added fats. Avoid hydrogenated (trans) fats, and use only small amounts of butter. Instead go for healthy oils, including sesame, walnut, and olive oil. For safety, use only olive or coconut oil for high-temperature cooking.

8.   Don't light up after a meal. Smoking cigarettes can aggravate hot flashes and night sweats and can bring on an earlier menopause. If you do smoke, try to pace yourself between cigarettes and cut down gradually until you can manage to quit the habit altogether. If you have been smoking for some time, you might need to be accountable during your withdrawal phase. Consider joining a smoking cessation program or seeing your doctor for some interim help.

9.   Finally, don't go shopping on an empty stomach, or you may be tempted to fill your basket with those high-fat, processed foods you are trying to avoid.

Below I offer quick options for meals and then go on to specify complete menus: four weeks' worth for omnivores and two weeks' worth for vegetarians and vegans. You don't have to eat everything on these menus; it's fine to limit your choices to a few selections, but make sure you stick to the rules and make your choices from these suggestions.

All the recommendations below are gluten-free. The notation (v) indicates items suitable for vegetarians; (vv) indicates items suitable for vegans. An asterisk indicates that a recipe is provided in the recipe section starting on page 187.

Quick Options
Breakfast

- Phyto muesli* with soy milk and chopped fresh fruit (vv)
- Fresh fruit salad* with soy yogurt and 1 tablespoon flaxseeds (vv)
- Chopped apple, almonds, flaxseeds, and honey with soy yogurt (vv)
- Banana and mixed berry smoothie (mixed berries and soy milk blended with ice) (vv)
- Rice cakes with organic nut butter or pure fruit spread (vv)
- Cornflakes with phyto sprinkle*, raisins, and chopped nuts (vv)
- Cornflakes with chopped banana and soy milk (vv)
- Scrambled eggs, grilled mushrooms, and tomatoes with rice cake (v)

- Two poached eggs on gluten-free toast with mushrooms and tomatoes (v)
- Boiled egg with rice cakes, corn crispbread, or gluten-free toast (v)

Lunch

- Raw vegetables (crudités) with dips such as hummus* and guacamole (vv)
- Refried soybeans with corn tacos (vv)
- Omelet with salad (v)
- Spicy soybeans*on gluten-free toast (vv)
- Stir-fried tofu and mixed vegetables with rice (vv)
- Soup (your choice) with gluten-free bread (vv)
- Rice salad with pumpkin seeds, sunflower seeds, and nuts (vv)
- Fruit and nut compote with soy yogurt (vv)
- Scrambled tofu* with gluten-free bread or baked potato (vv)
- Soy and buckwheat pancakes with refried soybeans (vv)
- Grilled tempeh with salad (vv)
- Bean tacos with salad (vv)
- Tempeh kebab with gluten-free pita bread (vv)
- Sesame tofu with salad (vv)
- Gluten-free soy and flaxseed bread with soy cheese and salad (vv)
- Rice cakes with almond butter and salad (vv)

Dinner

- Tofu kebabs with satay sauce, stir-fried vegetables, and rice (vv)
- Tofu risotto (vv)
- Lamb kebabs with vegetables and rice
- Salmon steaks with orange ginger sauce and vegetables
- Refried beans with rice, corn chips, and avocado (vv)
- Stir-fried tofu and vegetables with rice noodles (vv)
- Tofu burgers with salad and a baked potato (vv)
- Avocado with tuna, salad, and a baked potato
- Grilled lamb chop with rosemary, vegetables, and new potatoes

- Chicken kebabs with tamari and ginger dressing
- Spinach gratin with a baked potato (v)
- Noodles in spicy sesame sauce with edamame beans (vv)
- Cauliflower cheese with a baked potato (v)
- Sesame tofu with salad and a baked potato (vv)

Snacking

Depending on your weight goals and appetite, snacks and desserts are optional. I've included snack suggestions in the sample menus. If you are still menstruating, you need more nutrients in the week before your period: your calorie requirements increase by about five hundred calories per day. A wholesome midmorning and midafternoon snack might help meet your needs.

On the other hand, as our metabolic rate slows down in midlife, many women find it harder to avoid unwanted weight gain. If you enjoy snacking, you may need to reduce the portion sizes of your main meals so that you don't pile on the pounds. Also, keep in mind that adding soy products and flaxseeds to your diet may increase your calorie intake; adjust portion sizes as necessary to compensate.

Sample Menus for Omnivores
Week 1

Day 1

Breakfast
- Polenta porridge*
- Almonds, whole or sliced
- 2 tablespoons organic golden flaxseeds
- Chopped banana

Lunch
- Cauliflower soup*
- Rice or corn cakes
- Edamame beans

Dinner
- Grilled chicken with almonds
- Green beans
- Sweet corn
- Baked potato

Dessert
- Cinnamon-flavored rhubarb with soy yogurt

Snacks
- Dried apricots
- Almond cookie

Day 2

Breakfast
- Soy yogurt or soy milk
- Apple, chopped
- Sunflower seeds, pumpkin seeds, and chopped pecans
- 2 tablespoons organic golden flaxseeds

Lunch
- Scrambled tofu*
- Mixed green salad

Dinner
- Grilled polenta with vegetables
- Brown rice

Dessert
- Prune and tofu whip*

Snacks
- Orange
- Slice of phyto fruit loaf*

Day 3

Breakfast
- Phyto muesli* with soy milk
- Pear, chopped
- 2 tablespoons organic golden flaxseeds

Lunch
- Baked potato
- Edamame beans
- Green salad
- Apple

Dinner
- Pan-fried chicken
- Brown rice
- Sweet corn
- Broccoli

Dessert
- Apple-cinnamon muffin*

Snacks
- Banana
- Mixed unsalted nuts

Day 4

Breakfast
- Banana and rice pancakes* with soy yogurt, golden flaxseeds, and chopped fresh fruit

Lunch
- Spanish omelet*
- Salad of choice
- Apple

Dinner
- Ginger salmon*
- New potatoes
- Peas
- Carrots

Dessert
- Blueberry and tofu brûlée*

Snacks
- Pear
- Rice cakes with nut butter

Day 5

Breakfast
>   Polenta porridge*
>   Dried apricots
>   Almonds
>   2 tablespoons organic golden flaxseeds

Lunch
>   Vegetable soup
>   Soy or corn bread
>   Small piece of cheese
>   Apple

Dinner
>   Tuna steak
>   Beet, apple, and celery salad*
>   Steamed or boiled new potatoes

Dessert
>   Dried fruit compote* with soy yogurt

Snacks
>   Banana
>   Edamame beans

Day 6

Breakfast
>   Phyto fruit loaf*
>   Banana smoothie* with phyto
>   sprinkle*

Lunch
>   Baked potatoes with spicy soybeans*
>   or edamame beans
>   Coleslaw

Dinner
>   Fish with sweet soy sauce over
>   spinach*
>   Cauliflower
>   Carrots

Dessert
>   Passion fruit fool*

Snacks
>   Almond cookie
>   Edamame beans

Day 7

Breakfast
>   Phyto muesli* with soy milk
>   Chopped pear
>   2 tablespoons organic golden flaxseeds

Lunch
>   Gluten-free soy and flaxseed bread
>   Avocado
>   Apple and peanut salad*

Dinner
>   Nutty tofu rice*
>   Green salad

Dessert
>   Soufflé pancakes with strawberries*

Snacks
>   Phyto fix bar*
>   Edamame beans

Week 2

Day 1

Breakfast
Phyto muesli* with soy milk
Chopped pear
2 tablespoons organic golden flaxseeds

Lunch
Cauliflower soup*
Gluten-free bread
Apple

Dinner
Soba noodle and chicken soup*
Green beans
Sweet corn

Dessert
Banana rice*

Snacks
Edamame beans
Fruit bar*

Day 2

Breakfast
Scrambled tofu*
Organic raisins
Pecans
1 tablespoon organic golden flaxseeds

Lunch
Bean tacos with green salad
Apple

Dinner
Preserved-lemon risotto with salmon,
    artichokes, and asparagus*
Zucchini
Carrots

Dessert
Dried fruit compote* with soy yogurt

Snacks
Brazil nuts
Dried apricots

Day 3

Breakfast
Puffed rice cereal with soy milk
Chopped banana
Chopped pecans
Phyto sprinkle*

Lunch
Red lentil and coconut mash*
Brown rice

Dinner
Roast chicken
Roasted eggplant
Roast potatoes
Carrots
Cabbage

Dessert
Fresh fruit salad* with flaxseeds and
    soy yogurt

Snacks
Dried apricots
Almonds

Day 4

Breakfast
- Polenta porridge*
- Almonds
- Dried apricots
- Phyto sprinkle*

Lunch
- Scrambled tofu* on gluten-free toast
- Mixed salad
- Apple

Dinner
- Lamb stir-fry with fresh vegetables
- Rice noodles

Dessert
- Prune and tofu whip*

Snacks
- Banana
- Edamame beans

Day 5

Breakfast
- Cornflakes with soy milk
- Chopped banana
- Almonds
- Phyto sprinkle*
- 2 tablespoons organic golden flaxseeds

Lunch
- Baked potatoes with spicy soybeans*
  - or edamame beans
- Green salad

- Apple

Dinner
- Nutty tofu rice*
- Sweet potato salad*

Dessert
- Banana rice*

Snacks
- Fruit bar*
- Pear

Day 6

Breakfast
- Scrambled tofu*
- Slice of gluten-free toast

Lunch
- Carrot soup
- Soy or corn bread
- Edamame bean salad

Dinner
- Green chicken curry*
- Rice
- Popadam

Dessert
- Passion fruit fool*

Snacks
- Phyto fix bar*
- Edamame beans

Day 7

Breakfast
- Soy yogurt
- Chopped fresh fruit
- Almonds and pecans
- 2 tablespoons organic golden flaxseeds

Lunch
- Hummus* and crudités
- Corn chips
- Apple

Dinner
- Noodles with chicken
- Green beans
- Sweet corn

Dessert
- Rhubarb and ginger mousse*

Snacks
- Brazil nuts
- Banana

Week 3

Day 1

Breakfast
- Polenta porridge*
- Dried apricots
- Chopped almonds
- 1 tablespoon organic golden flaxseeds

Lunch
- Soy and rice pancakes* with refried soybeans
- Green salad
- Pear

Dinner
- Fish with sweet soy sauce over spinach*
- Brown rice
- Green beans and carrots

Dessert
- Fresh fruit salad* sprinkled with 1 tablespoon organic golden flaxseeds

Snacks
- Blueberry and rhubarb smoothie*
- Rice cake with almond butter

Day 2

Breakfast
- Phyto muesli* with soy milk
- Chopped banana
- 2 tablespoons organic golden flaxseeds

Lunch
- Baked potatoes with spicy soybeans*
- Waldorf salad*

Dinner
- Polenta with grilled vegetables*
- Green salad

Dessert
- Banana and tofu cream*

Snacks
- Edamame beans
- Dried apricots

Day 3

Breakfast
> Cornflakes with soy milk
> Chopped banana
> Almonds
> Phyto sprinkle* with additional golden
>   flaxseeds

Lunch
> Scrambled tofu* on gluten-free toast
> Green salad

Dinner
> Grilled tuna steak
> New potatoes
> Carrots
> Broccoli

Dessert
> Dried fruit compote* with soy yogurt,
>   sprinkled with 1 tablespoon
>   organic golden flaxseeds

Snacks
> Apple
> Sunflower seeds and pumpkin seeds

Day 4

Breakfast
> Soy yogurt
> Berries
> Almonds
> 2 tablespoons organic golden flaxseeds
> Half of an apple-cinnamon muffin*

Lunch
> Hummus* with crudités
> Corn chips
> Pear

Dinner
> Nutty tofu rice*
> Beet, apple, and celery salad*

Dessert
> Dried fruit compote* with soy yogurt

Snacks
> Coconut cookie
> Banana

Day 5

Breakfast
Scrambled tofu*
Slice of gluten-free toast

Lunch
Niçoise salad with tofu–soy milk
     dressing*
Apple

Dinner
Rosemary arancini*
Sweet corn
Broccoli

Dessert
Phyto fix bar*

Snacks
Banana smoothie*
Edamame beans

Day 6

Breakfast
Phyto muesli*
Soy yogurt
Chopped banana
2 tablespoons organic golden flaxseeds

Lunch
Lentil soup
Corn bread
Apple and peanut salad*

Dinner
Ginger salmon*
Green salad
New potatoes

Dessert
Passion fruit fool*

Snacks
Blueberry and rhubarb smoothie*
Apple

Day 7

Breakfast
Banana and rice pancakes* with soy
     yogurt and honey, sprinkled
     with 1 tablespoon organic golden
     flaxseeds

Lunch
Cauliflower soup*
Corn bread
Pear

Dinner
Nutty brussels sprout stir-fry*
Brown rice
Green salad

Dessert
Phyto fruit loaf*

Snacks
Apple
Almonds

Week 4

Day 1

Breakfast
- Cornflakes with soy milk
- Dried apricots
- Almonds, whole or flaked
- 2 tablespoons organic golden flaxseeds

Lunch
- Hummus*
- Corn chips
- Green salad

Dinner
- Red lentil and coconut mash*
- Baked potato
- Broccoli

Dessert
- Banana and tofu cream*

Snacks
- Phyto fix bar*
- Brazil nuts

Day 2

Breakfast
- Puffed rice cereal with soy milk
- Chopped banana
- Chopped pecans
- 2 tablespoons organic golden flaxseeds

Lunch
- Scrambled tofu*
- Salad
- Pear

Dinner
- Lamb stir-fry with vegetables
- Rice

Dessert
- Dried fruit compote* with soy yogurt

Snacks
- Phyto fruit loaf*
- Pear

Day 3

Breakfast
- Phyto muesli* with soy milk
- Chopped banana
- 2 tablespoons organic golden flaxseeds

Lunch
- Guacamole with crudités
- Corn tacos
- Apple

Dinner
- Preserved-lemon risotto with salmon, artichokes, and asparagus*
- Sweet potato salad*

Dessert
- Banana rice*
- Dried apricots

Snacks
- Edamame beans
- Mixed unsalted nuts

Day 4

Breakfast
Soy yogurt
Chopped banana
Almonds, whole or sliced
2 tablespoons organic golden flaxseeds

Lunch
Hummus*
Rice crispbreads or corn chips
Green salad

Dinner
Green chicken curry*
Green beans
Carrots
Brown rice

Dessert
Rhubarb and ginger mousse*

Snacks
Edamame beans
Phyto fix bar*

Day 5

Breakfast
Polenta porridge*
Chopped dried apricots
Sliced almonds
1 tablespoon organic golden flaxseeds

Lunch
Baked potatoes with spicy soybeans*
    or edamame beans
Green salad
Banana

Dinner
Nutty brussels sprout stir-fry*
Sweet corn
Green beans

Dessert
Fresh fruit salad* with golden flaxseeds

Snacks
Phyto fix bar*
Apple

Day 6

Breakfast
Phyto muesli* with soy milk
Chopped banana
2 tablespoons organic golden flaxseeds

Lunch
Baked potato with edamame beans
Green salad

Dinner
Tofu, bean, and herb stir-fry
Broccoli

Dessert
Apple-cinnamon muffin*

Snacks
Almonds
Edamame beans

Day 7

Breakfast
Soy yogurt
Chopped kiwifruit and banana
Almonds
Pumpkin seeds
2 tablespoons organic golden flaxseeds

Lunch
Tuna sandwich on gluten-free soy and
flaxseed bread
Apple and peanut salad*

Dinner
Pan-fried chicken
Stir-fried vegetables with brown rice

Dessert
Stewed apple and blackberries with
soy yogurt

Snacks
Banana bread*
Pear

Sample Menus for Vegetarians
Week 1

Day 1

Breakfast
Scrambled tofu* with tomatoes
Slice gluten-free toast

Lunch
Hummus* with crudités and edamame
beans
Corn chips
Apple

Dinner
Tofu and bean stir-fry with vegetables
Brown rice

Dessert
Rhubarb and ginger mousse*

Snacks
Apple-cinnamon muffin*
Pear

Day 2

Breakfast
Polenta porridge*
2 tablespoons organic golden flaxseeds
Organic raisins, dried apricots

Lunch
Cauliflower soup*
Corn bread

Dinner
Red lentil and coconut mash*
Brown rice
Broccoli

Dessert
Prune and tofu whip*

Snacks
Apple-cinnamon muffin*
Almonds

Day 3

Breakfast
Dried fruit compote* with soy yogurt
Sliced almonds
2 tablespoons organic golden flaxseeds

Lunch
Guacamole
Corn or rice chips
Beet, apple, and celery salad*

Dinner
Spanish omelet*
Sautéed potatoes
Green salad

Dessert
Blueberry and tofu brûlée*

Snacks
Banana
Edamame beans

Day 4

Breakfast
Cornflakes and/or puffed rice cereal
    with soy milk
Sliced almonds and chopped pecans
Dried apricots
2 tablespoons organic golden flaxseeds

Lunch
Rosemary arancini*
Green salad

Dinner
Nutty brussels sprout stir-fry*
Brown rice
Carrots

Dessert
Passion fruit fool*

Snacks
Soy nuts
Apple

Day 5

Breakfast
Poached egg or (for vegans) blueberry
    and rhubarb smoothie
Gluten-free soy and flaxseed bread,
    toasted (with almond butter for
    vegans)

Lunch
Apple and peanut salad*
Half an avocado

Dinner
Nutty tofu rice*
Zucchini

Dessert
Blueberry and tofu brûlée*

Snacks
Soy yogurt
Dried apricots

Day 6

Breakfast
Soy yogurt
Chopped banana and pear
2 tablespoons organic golden flaxseeds
Rice cakes and marmalade

Lunch
Baked potato with hummus* and
    edamame beans
Root vegetable salad*

Dinner
Polenta with grilled vegetables*
Sweet potato salad*

Dessert
Banana and rice pancakes*

Snacks
Pear
Edamame beans

Day 7

Breakfast
Phyto muesli* with soy milk
Chopped pear
2 tablespoons organic golden flaxseeds

Lunch
Baked potato with hummus* and
    edamame beans
Green salad
Apple

Dinner
Tofu and bean stir-fry with mixed
    vegetables
Rice noodles

Dessert
Passion fruit fool*

Snacks
Fruit bar*
Pear

Week 2

Day 1

Breakfast
Polenta porridge*
Chopped banana
Almonds, whole or sliced
2 tablespoons organic golden flaxseeds

Lunch
Cauliflower soup*
Gluten-free soy and flaxseed toast
Apple

Dinner
Nutty brussels sprout stir-fry*
Apple and peanut salad*

Dessert
Banana rice*

Snacks
Pear
Soy nuts

Day 2

Breakfast
  Polenta porridge*
  Chopped banana
  Dried apricots
  2 tablespoons organic golden flaxseeds

Lunch
  Baked potato with edamame beans
  Green salad
  Apple

Dinner
  Nutty tofu rice*
  Carrots
  Green beans

Dessert
  Blueberry and tofu brûlée*

Snacks
  Pear
  Edamame beans

Day 3

Breakfast
  Cornflakes with soy milk
  Almonds
  Blueberries
  2 tablespoons organic golden flaxseeds

Lunch
  Scrambled tofu*
  Cornbread
  Apple

Dinner
  Rosemary arancini*
  Apple and peanut salad*

Dessert
  Passion fruit fool*

Snacks
  Phyto fruit loaf*
  Pear

Day 4

Breakfast
  Banana and rice pancakes* with soy
    yogurt, sprinkled with 1 table-
    spoon organic golden flaxseeds

Lunch
  Cauliflower soup*
  Gluten-free soy and flaxseed bread
  Pear

Dinner
  Red lentil and coconut mash*
  Basmati rice
  Stir-fried vegetables
  Popadam

Dessert
  Banana rice*

Snacks
  Dried apricots
  Edamame beans

Day 5

Breakfast
Cornflakes with soy milk
Dried apricots
Pumpkin seeds and pecans
2 tablespoons organic golden flaxseeds

Lunch
Scrambled tofu*
Gluten-free bread
Mixed salad
Apple

Dinner
Polenta with grilled vegetables*
Apple and peanut salad*
Green beans

Dessert
Passion fruit fool*

Snacks
Phyto fix bar*
Pear

Day 6

Breakfast
Mixed berry smoothie* with 2 tablespoons organic golden flaxseeds

Lunch
Baked potato with hummus* and
edamame beans
Root vegetable salad*

Dinner
Tofu and bean stir-fry with vegetables
Baked potato

Dessert
Blueberry and tofu brûlée*

Snacks
Phyto fix bar*
Apple

Day 7

Breakfast
Polenta porridge*
Chopped banana
Sliced almonds
2 tablespoons organic golden flaxseeds

Lunch
Avocado
Beet, apple, and celery salad*
Melon

Dinner
Nutty tofu rice*
Green beans
Carrots

Dessert
Prune and tofu whip*

Snacks
Banana
Edamame beans

Chapter 12

RECIPES FOR A HEALTHIER, HAPPIER YOU

Soy- and phyto-rich food doesn't need to be bland or boring. Here is a selection of quick and easy recipes brimming with these essential nutrients and guaranteed to tempt your taste buds.

 BREAKFAST AND BRUNCH DISHES

Phyto Muesli

Makes 12 servings

16 ounces (16 cups) puffed rice
8 ounces (8 cups) cornflakes
4 ounces (½ cup) chopped almonds
4 ounces (½ cup) pumpkin seeds
4 ounces (½ cup) chopped pecans
4 ounces (½ cup) sesame seeds
4 ounces (½ cup) pine nuts

4 ounces (⅓ cup) organic flaxseeds
6 ounces (⅔ cup) organic raisins
4 ounces organic unsulfured dried apricots, chopped

In a large bowl, mix all the ingredients together. Store in a sealed container. Serve with a cup of soy yogurt or soy milk and fresh fruit. To relieve constipation, sprinkle additional flaxseeds over your morning muesli.

Phyto Fruit Loaf

Makes two 1-pound loaves

5 ounces (¾ cup) soy flour
4 ounces (½ cup) buckwheat flour
4 ounces (½ cup) flaxseeds (whole)
4 ounces (½ cup) ground almonds
2 ounces (¼ cup) sesame seeds
2 ounces (¼ cup) sunflower seeds
10 ounces (1⅓ cups) unsulfured dried fruit
2 level tablespoons unrefined sugar
1 teaspoon ground nutmeg
1 teaspoon mixed spice
1 tablespoon ground cinnamon
Two 1-inch pieces fresh ginger root, chopped
2 teaspoons gluten-free baking powder
30 fluid ounces (3¾ cups) soy milk

Mix all the dry ingredients in a large bowl, then stir in the soy milk. Leave the mixture to stand for 1 hour. Spoon into two 8½ × 4¼ -inch (1-pound) greased loaf pans. Bake at 350 °F (180 °C) for 1 to 1½ hours until firm on top. Transfer onto a wire rack and allow the loaves to cool. Slice and serve with butter, cheese, or fruit or nut spreads.

Polenta Porridge

Makes 2 servings

3 ounces (½ cup) fine-ground instant polenta
10 fluid ounces (1¼ cups) soy milk
16 fluid ounces (2 cups) water

Combine the soy milk and water. Bring two-thirds of the liquid to the boil over low to medium heat. Gradually add the polenta and stir constantly. When the mixture starts to get thick, add the rest of the liquid and keep stirring until the polenta no longer feels grainy, which should take 3–5 minutes. Top with fruit, phyto sprinkle (see recipe below), and soy yogurt to taste.

Scrambled Tofu

Makes 4 servings

1 tablespoon soy oil
1 small onion, finely chopped
1 carrot, finely chopped
1 potato, diced
20 ounces tofu, diced
1½ teaspoons ground turmeric
½ teaspoon ground black pepper
2 tomatoes, halved
4 mushrooms
4 slices gluten-free toast

Heat the oil in a large frying pan over low heat. Add the onion and cook, stirring occasionally, for 2–3 minutes, until it starts to turn golden. Add the carrot and potato and cook, stirring frequently, for a further 10 minutes until the vegetables are slightly soft. Stir in the tofu, turmeric, and black pepper, cover with a lid, and cook for 5 minutes, until the mixture is heated through and has absorbed all the flavors.

Meanwhile, preheat the broiler to medium. Broil the tomatoes and mushrooms until their tops are slightly golden.

Serve the scrambled tofu hot, with the tomatoes, mushrooms, and toast.

Phyto Sprinkle

This excellent source of phytoestrogens can easily be incorporated into your daily diet. Sprinkle 1–2 tablespoons over breakfast cereals, salads, and desserts, and add it to bread and cake recipes.

Makes about 2 cups

4 ounces (½ cup) almonds
4 ounces (½ cup) sunflower seeds
4 ounces (½ cup) pumpkin seeds
4 ounces (½ cup) golden flaxseeds

In a blender, process all the ingredients to a coarse consistency. Store in a sealed container in the refrigerator.

Spanish Omelet

Makes 6 servings

3 tablespoons olive oil
3 small red potatoes (about 12 ounces), peeled and sliced
1 medium red bell pepper, cut into ½-inch strips
1 red onion, halved and thinly sliced
Salt and freshly ground black pepper
1 tablespoon fresh oregano leaves (or 1 teaspoon dried oregano)
6 eggs
4 fluid ounces (½ cup) soy milk

Heat the oil in a large ovenproof, nonstick frying pan over medium heat. Add the potatoes and the red bell pepper. Cover the pan and cook for 10 minutes, stirring occasionally. Add the onion. Cover and cook for a further 10 minutes, stirring occasionally. Season with salt and pepper. Add the oregano.

Preheat the broiler. Whisk together the eggs and soy milk and pour the mixture over the vegetables in the pan. Cover and cook over medium heat for 5 minutes, or until the base is golden. Place the pan under the preheated broiler and broil until the top is golden. Slice the omelet and serve with a salad of lettuce, olives, and shaved parmesan.

Banana Bread

Makes one 1-pound loaf

2 ripe bananas, peeled
4 fluid ounces (½ cup) vegetable oil
2 eggs, beaten
3¼ ounces (½ cup) brown sugar, lightly packed
4 fluid ounces (½ cup) soy milk
8 ounces (1¼ cup) coconut flour
3 ounces (½ cup) spelt flour
1 teaspoon gluten-free baking powder
1 teaspoon ground cinnamon
2¼ ounces (½ cup) roasted hazelnuts
4 ounces (½ cup) chopped dried banana
4¼ ounces (½ cup) fresh raspberries

Preheat the oven to 350°F (180°C). Lightly grease an 8½ × 4¼-inch (1-pound) loaf pan. In a medium-sized mixing bowl, mash the bananas, then whisk them together with the oil, eggs, sugar, and soy milk. Sift in the flours, baking powder, and cinnamon. Gently fold in the hazelnuts, dried banana, and raspberries. Pour into the loaf pan and bake for 1 hour, or until a skewer inserted into the center comes out clean. Turn out onto a rack to cool. Slice and serve with soy cream cheese and honey.

Apple-Cinnamon Muffins

Makes 12 muffins

4 ounces tofu, crumbled
4 ounces (½ cup) grated apple
5 fluid ounces soy milk
2 eggs
2 ounces (¼ cup) potato flour
2 ounces (¼ cup) cornmeal
2 ounces (¼ cup) rice flour
2 ounces (¼ cup) soy flour
1 teaspoon unrefined sugar
1 tablespoon ground cinnamon
1 teaspoon baking soda
1 teaspoon cream of tartar
1 tablespoon olive oil
Soy margarine or butter for greasing pan

Preheat the oven to 425°F (220°C). Beat the tofu, apple, milk, and eggs to a smooth puree. Mix the dry ingredients with the olive oil, then fold the mixture into the puree. (Do not overmix or leave the batter to stand, otherwise the muffins will be heavy.) Grease a 12-cup muffin pan with the soy margarine and spoon in the batter. Bake for 12–15 minutes. Remove the muffins from the pan and let cool.

Soy and Rice Pancakes

Makes 12 pancakes (4 servings)

2 ounces (¼ cup) soy flour
2 ounces (¼ cup) rice flour
1 small egg
10 fluid ounces (1¼ cups) soy milk
Soy oil for greasing pan

In a mixing bowl, beat the flours, egg, and milk into a thin batter. Wipe a small nonstick frying pan with a little soy oil and place over medium heat. Once the oil is hot (sprinkle a few drops of water on the pan; they should sizzle), pour about 2 tablespoons of the batter into the pan and swirl it around to cover the base of the pan. Cook for 1 minute, until golden underneath, then flip the pancake and cook the other side. Set aside. Repeat with the rest of the batter.

Banana and Rice Pancakes

Makes 12 pancakes (4 servings)

2 ounces (¼ cup) rice flakes
2 ounces (¼ cup) soy flour
1 ounce (⅛ cup) rice flour
1 tablespoon baking powder
6 fluid ounces (¾ cup) soy milk
2 bananas, thinly sliced

Combine the dry ingredients in a bowl. Stir in the milk to make a thin batter. Fold in the sliced banana. Pour 2 tablespoons of the mixture into a lightly oiled nonstick frying pan. Cook until bubbles appear on the surface, then flip the pancake and cook for about 1 minute more. Serve warm with pure maple syrup, soy yogurt, and fresh fruit.

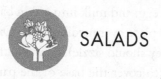

SALADS

Apple and Peanut Salad

Makes 4 servings

4 red apples
Juice of half a lemon
½ cucumber, thickly sliced and quartered, peeled if you prefer
6 celery sticks, chopped
1 bunch green onions, sliced in rounds
3 ounces (½ cup) unsalted peanuts (or other nuts)

Core and roughly chop the apples. Dip them in the lemon juice to slow discoloration. Combine all the ingredients, toss with the dressing of your choice, and serve.

Sweet Potato Salad

Makes 4 servings

1 pound (about 3 cups) sweet potato, cubed and steamed
1 tablespoon soy oil
3 tablespoons lemon juice
1–2 cloves garlic, crushed
1 tablespoon parsley, chopped
1 tablespoon fresh basil, chopped
1 tablespoon fresh chives, chopped
1 tablespoon spring onion, chopped

Combine all ingredients. Season with black pepper.

Niçoise Salad with Tofu–Soy Milk Dressing

Makes 4 servings

SALAD

3 eggs
8 small potatoes, halved
10 ounces tuna steak
Olive oil spray
7 ounces (¾ cup) thin green beans
7 ounces (¾ cup) grape tomatoes, halved
4 ounces small black olives, pitted
1 baby romaine lettuce, leaves separated

DRESSING

5½ ounces (¾ cup) silken tofu
4 fluid ounces (½ cup) soy milk
1 clove garlic, chopped
1 teaspoon Dijon mustard
2 tablespoons lime juice

Place the eggs in a small saucepan and cover with cold water. Bring the water to a boil, then reduce the heat to low and simmer for 5 minutes. Place the eggs in cold water until cool, then peel, slice, and set them aside.

Cook the potatoes in boiling salted water for 10 minutes, or until just tender. Lightly spray the tuna with olive oil, then chargrill for 2–3 minutes on each side, or until just cooked. Flake the fish into pieces using two forks. Blanch the beans in boiling salted water for 1 minute, then refresh in cold water. Toss the eggs, potatoes, tuna, beans, tomatoes, olives, and lettuce together in a large bowl.

To make the dressing, combine all the ingredients in a blender and process until smooth. Season with salt and freshly ground black pepper. Drizzle over salad.

Beet, Apple, and Celery Salad

Makes 4 servings

1 large beet, cooked and cubed
1 apple, sliced and cored but not peeled
1 stick celery, diced
1 tablespoon chopped walnuts
1 tablespoon French dressing,, or dressing of your choice

Combine all ingredients.

Waldorf Salad

Makes 4 servings

2 ounces walnuts, coarsely chopped
1 head curly endive, chopped
2 apples, chopped
2 sticks celery, sliced
1 tablespoon organic golden flaxseeds
Freshly ground black pepper
Salad dressing of your choice

Combine the walnuts, endive, apples, celery, and flaxseeds. Season with black pepper and dressing.

Root Vegetable Salad

Makes 4 servings

4 ounces celery root (celeriac), chopped or grated
6 ounces carrots, chopped or grated
4 ounces parsnips, chopped or grated
3 ounces cooked beets, chopped

Combine the celery root, carrots, and parsnips. Sprinkle the chopped beets on top of the salad. Sprinkle with fresh black pepper and drizzle with your favorite dressing.

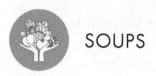

SOUPS

Corn Chowder with Garlic Shrimp

Makes 2 servings

3 tablespoons butter
1 small onion, finely diced
3 garlic cloves, finely chopped
1 medium potato, peeled and diced
2 cobs fresh corn, shucked (or 1 cup frozen or canned corn kernels,
    drained and rinsed)
1 celery stick, diced
24 fluid ounces (3 cups) soy milk
1 cup vegetable stock
Freshly ground black pepper
1 tablespoon olive oil
9 ounces peeled shrimp
½ cup fresh flat-leaf parsley leaves, chopped

Heat the butter in a large saucepan until it foams. Add the onion and one-third of the garlic. Cook over medium heat for 2 minutes. Add the potato and cook for 2 minutes. Add the corn, celery, and soy milk. Bring to a boil, then reduce heat and simmer for 10 minutes or until the vegetables are just tender. Add the vegetable stock and pepper.

Heat the oil in a frying pan. Add the remaining garlic and the shrimp. Cook over medium-high heat for 2 minutes, or until the shrimp turn opaque. Remove the chowder from the heat and stir in the parsley. Spoon into bowls and serve topped with the shrimp.

Soba Noodle and Chicken Soup

Makes 4 servings

64 fluid ounces (8 cups) chicken stock
2 cloves garlic, chopped

1 tablespoon grated fresh ginger root
2 stalks lemongrass, finely chopped
2 boneless skinless chicken breasts
1 cup shiitake mushrooms
1 head broccoli, cut into florets
9 ounces (1 package) dried soba noodles (or rice noodles)

Place the stock, garlic, ginger, and lemongrass in a large saucepan and bring to a boil. Add the chicken breasts and simmer for 8–10 minutes, or until cooked through. Add the mushrooms and broccoli and simmer for a further 3-5 minutes. Meanwhile, cook noodles in plenty of boiling water until al dente, then drain and divide into serving bowls. Remove chicken from soup and slice, then return it to the soup and stir. Ladle the soup over the noodles and serve.

Cauliflower Soup

Makes 4 servings

2 ounces (¼ cup) soy margarine
4 ounces (½ cup) soy flour
8 fluid ounces (1 cup) soy milk
30 fluid ounces (3¾ cups) vegetable stock
1 large cauliflower, broken into florets
1 teaspoon dried chervil
Freshly ground black pepper, to taste

Melt the margarine in a large saucepan. Add the flour and cook for 1 minute, stirring constantly. Remove the pan from the heat and gradually stir in the milk and stock until the mixture is smooth and thick enough to coat the back of a spoon. Add the cauliflower and chervil. Season with the pepper. Simmer the soup gently for 15 minutes, until the cauliflower is just tender. Using an immersion blender, process the soup to a smooth puree. Serve piping hot with crusty bread.

MAIN DISHES

Fish with Sweet Soy Sauce over Spinach

Makes 2 servings

Two 6-ounce white fish fillets, such as mahimahi, halibut, or Chilean sea bass
1 teaspoon sesame oil
2 tablespoons gluten-free sweet soy sauce
8 fluid ounces (1 cup) chicken stock
14 large handfuls spinach leaves, washed and destalked
2 cloves garlic, chopped
1 red chile, chopped
1 tablespoon gluten-free tamari

Sear the fish on both sides in a hot pan with sesame oil and chopped garlic, adding a little stock if necessary to keep the fish moist. Add the soy sauce and ½ cup of the stock. Reduce until the sauce forms a glaze for the fish. Meanwhile, stir-fry the spinach with the garlic, chile, tamari, and remaining stock until the spinach wilts, then place the mixture in individual bowls and top with the fish.

Preserved-Lemon Risotto with Salmon, Artichokes, and Asparagus

Makes 6 servings

24 fluid ounces (3 cups) soy milk
16 fluid ounces (2 cups) chicken stock
3 tablespoons butter
1 tablespoon olive oil
1 small red onion, thinly sliced
2 garlic cloves, finely chopped
Half of a preserved lemon, chopped

11½ ounces (1½ cups) arborio rice
Salt and freshly ground black pepper
10½ ounces marinated artichoke hearts, sliced
1 bunch asparagus, trimmed
14 ounces salmon fillet
Olive oil, for rubbing

Place the soy milk and stock in a saucepan and bring just to a boil. Reduce the heat to a simmer. Heat the butter and oil in another saucepan over medium heat. Add the onion and garlic and cook until soft, stirring often. Add preserved lemon and rice. Stir over medium heat for 1–2 minutes, until the rice grains are slightly transparent.

Slowly add the soy milk and stock to the rice, a ladleful at a time, stirring constantly after each addition until the liquid is completely absorbed. Continue stirring until the rice is just cooked (with just a little resistance when you bite into a rice grain). This process should take about 20 minutes. Season with salt and pepper. Stir in the artichokes. Set the risotto aside while you cook the asparagus and salmon.

Wash the asparagus and steam it for 5 minutes, then drain it and set aside. While the asparagus is cooking, rub the salmon with olive oil and season it with salt and pepper. Cook the salmon in a frying pan over medium heat for 2–3 minutes on each side or until cooked through. Place it on a board and pull it apart into flakes with two forks. Serve the risotto topped with the salmon and asparagus.

Green Chicken Curry

Makes 6 servings

1 tablespoon vegetable oil
1 pound 2 ounces chicken tenderloins, cut into strips
2–3 tablespoons green Thai curry paste
5 fluid ounces (1 small can) coconut cream
8 fluid ounces (1 cup) soy milk
1 tablespoon fish sauce
8 ounces (1 can) sliced bamboo shoots, rinsed
4½ ounces (¾ cup) frozen or canned baby corn

4 ounces sugar snap peas, trimmed
A handful of fresh Thai basil leaves
Steamed jasmine rice

Heat the oil in a frying pan or wok. Add the chicken and curry paste and cook over medium heat, stirring constantly, for 5 minutes, or until the chicken is browned all over. Add
the coconut cream, soy milk, and fish sauce. Bring to a boil, stirring occasionally. Add the
bamboo shoots and corn. Cook until the corn is just tender. Remove the pan from the heat
and stir in the snow peas and basil. Serve with rice.

Hummus

Makes about 1½ cups

8 ounces (1 cup) dried chickpeas
5½ ounces (½ cup) sesame seeds
2 tablespoons tahini
2 tablespoons soy oil
5 cloves garlic
Juice of 3 lemons
Paprika, to taste (optional)

Soak the chickpeas overnight in water. Drain and rinse. Place the chickpeas in a pot of
water and bring to a boil, then simmer gently for 1½–2 hours, or until tender. Drain again.
In a blender or food processor, blend the sesame seeds, tahini, oil, garlic, and half the
lemon juice to a smooth puree. Gradually add the chickpeas and remaining lemon juice,
blending until smooth. If desired, add a pinch of paprika. Serve with crudités, corn chips,
or rice cakes.

Ginger Salmon

Makes 2 servings

2 medium salmon steaks
2 tablespoons lemon juice

One 1-inch cube fresh ginger root, peeled and finely chopped
Freshly ground black pepper, to taste

Preheat oven to 350°F (180°C). Place each salmon steak on a piece of foil. Top each steak with lemon juice and ginger and season with black pepper. Wrap each steak in foil and bake for 20 minutes. Serve with vegetables or salad.

Baked Potatoes with Spicy Soybeans

Makes 6 servings

10 ounces dried soybeans, washed and drained
3 bay leaves
2 tablespoons soy oil
2 cloves garlic, chopped
1 large onion, chopped
One 2-inch piece of cinnamon stick
10 ounces pureed tomatoes (passata)
5 fluid ounces molasses
5 fluid ounces prepared mustard
35 fluid ounces vegetable stock
6 large baking potatoes, scrubbed and pierced several times
2 tablespoons apple cider vinegar
1 tablespoon tamari

Wash the soybeans and soak overnight. Drain the beans, rinse well, and drain again before cooking.

Preheat the oven to 400°F (200°C). Heat the oil in a saucepan and sauté the garlic and onion until tender. Add the cinnamon stick and bay leaves and stir for 1 minute. Add the pureed tomatoes, molasses, mustard, and stock. Stir the mixture well and bring to the boil. Add the beans, bring to the boil again, then cover the pan, reduce the heat to low, and simmer gently for 2 hours, or until tender. Stir once during this time, adding more stock if necessary to keep the dish moist.

While the beans are cooking, bake the potatoes for about 1 hour 15 minutes, or until tender.

When the beans are done, remove the cinnamon stick and bay leaves. Stir in the vinegar and tamari. Remove the pot from the heat. The beans should be thick and the sauce richly flavored. Cut the potatoes open, spoon the beans over them, and serve immediately.

Rosemary Arancini

Makes 12

16 fluid ounces (2 cups) soy milk
16 fluid ounces (2 cups) chicken stock
3 tablespoons butter
1 onion, finely diced
1 clove garlic, crushed
8 ounces (1 cup) arborio rice
2 ounces fresh mozzarella cheese, cut into small cubes
Oil for deep-frying
2 eggs, beaten
8 ounces (1 cup) dry breadcrumbs
12 small sprigs fresh rosemary

Pour the soy milk and stock into a medium-sized saucepan and bring to a boil. Remove the pan from the heat. Heat the butter in a large saucepan. Add the onion and garlic and sauté over medium heat for 2–3 minutes, or until soft. Add the rice and stir for 1 minute, or until the rice grains are transparent. Add the liquid to the rice mixture one ladleful at a time, stirring constantly after each addition until all the liquid is absorbed. This process should take about 20–25 minutes. Set risotto aside to cool.

Divide the risotto into 12 equal portions and roll them into balls. Gently press your thumb into each ball and place a cube of mozzarella in the indentation, then pinch the risotto to enclose the cheese, and roll the balls again. Place the balls on a tray, cover, and refrigerate until required.

Heat the oil in a large frying pan until hot. (The oil is ready when a small cube of bread added to it turns golden.) Dip each risotto ball first into the beaten egg, then into the breadcrumbs. Spear each ball with a sprig of rosemary and deep-fry the balls, two at a time, until golden brown. Use a slotted spoon to transfer the cooked balls onto a paper towel. Serve warm.

Nutty Tofu Rice

Makes 4 servings

8 ounces brown rice
1 tablespoon sunflower oil
1 medium onion, chopped fine
1 clove garlic, chopped fine
1 red bell pepper, seeded and sliced
1 green bell pepper, seeded and sliced
2 ounces green beans, trimmed, strings removed, and cut into 1-inch pieces
4 ounces carrots, cut into matchsticks
4 ounces zucchini, thinly sliced
4 ounces broccoli, broken into florets, stalks sliced thin
8 ounces tofu
1 small seedless orange, peeled and sectioned
1 tablespoon sliced almonds
1 tablespoon fresh chopped parsley

Cook the rice according to package directions and set it aside. Heat the oil in a large frying pan. Add the onion, garlic, and the red and green bell peppers and sauté gently for 2–3 minutes. Steam the beans, carrots, zucchini, and broccoli for 5 minutes (or add them straight to the pan if you like your vegetables crunchy), then add to the other ingredients in the frying pan. Add the tofu, orange, almonds, parsley, and rice, and cook gently until dish is heated through. Serve immediately.

Red Lentil and Coconut Mash

Makes 4 servings

8 ounces red split lentils
4 ounces carrots, peeled and sliced

1 medium onion, finely chopped
1 clove garlic, crushed
1 teaspoon paprika
½ teaspoon ground ginger
1 bay leaf
16 fluid ounces (2 cups) water
1 tablespoon creamed coconut, finely chopped
2 tablespoons lemon juice
Ground black pepper

Wash the lentils and put them into a large saucepan with the carrots, onion, garlic, paprika, ginger, bay leaf, and water. Bring to the boil, skim to remove any scum, cover the pan, and simmer for 25–30 minutes, or until the water has been absorbed. Remove the bay leaf and mash the mixture into a smooth paste with a fork. Add the creamed coconut, lemon juice, and black pepper to taste. Serve hot with vegetables or rice.

Nutty Brussels Sprout Stir-Fry

Makes 4 servings

3 ounces unsalted shelled peanuts
1 medium orange, peeled and cut into sections
2 tablespoons sesame oil
Pinch of cayenne pepper
½ teaspoon ground cumin
2 thick spring onions, trimmed and sliced
1 garlic clove, thinly sliced
6 ounces brussels sprouts, trimmed and thinly sliced
1 red bell pepper, cored, seeded, and thinly sliced
2 tablespoons gluten-free soy sauce or tamari

Preheat the oven to 375°F (190°C). Place the peanuts in a baking dish and bake about 10 minutes, or until lightly roasted. Slice the orange sections crossways into triangles.

Heat the sesame oil in a wok or heavy frying pan. Add the cayenne pepper, cumin, spring onions, garlic, and brussels sprouts and toss in the oil for 1 minute. Add the roasted peanuts and red bell pepper, mix and continue to cook for 1 minute more. Add the orange pieces and soy sauce and stir-fry until all the vegetables are coated with sauce and the orange pieces are heated through. Serve immediately with rice or baked potatoes.

Polenta with Grilled Vegetables

Makes 4-6 servings

POLENTA

6 ounces (1 cup) polenta
8 ounces (1 cup) cold water (or vegetable broth)
24 fluid ounces (3 cups) boiling water
2 tablespoons butter, plus extra for grilling
Salt to taste

VEGETABLES

2 zucchini, halved lengthways and sliced thick
1 fennel bulb, trimmed and quartered lengthways
2 tomatoes, cored and sliced
1 eggplant, halved lengthways and sliced
1 red bell pepper, halved, seeded, and sliced
1 green bell pepper, halved, seeded, and sliced

VEGETABLE MARINADE

2 tablespoons olive oil
2 tablespoons red wine vinegar
2-3 tablespoons chopped parsley
2 garlic cloves, crushed
Salt and ground black pepper to taste

ALTERNATE MARINADE

2 tablespoons sunflower oil
2 tablespoons tamari or gluten-free soy sauce
1 tablespoon clear honey
2 teaspoons Dijon mustard
Salt and ground black pepper to taste

To make the vegetable marinade, combine the oil, vinegar, parsley, and garlic, and add salt, and pepper to taste. Add the vegetables, stir to coat them thoroughly, and refrigerate while you cook the polenta.

Put the polenta into a saucepan, cover with the measured cold water, and leave to stand for 5 minutes. Add the boiling salted water to the pan and bring it back to the boil, whisking for 5 minutes to ensure that there are no lumps. Simmer for a further 25 minutes, whisking every five minutes, until the polenta is smooth and thickened. Sprinkle a medium-sized (approximately 10 × 8.5-inch) baking dish with water. Stir the butter into the polenta and then spread the mixture into the dish to form a layer about ½ inch thick. Leave it to cool.

Remove the vegetables from the marinade and cook over a hot barbecue (or in a roasting pan under a broiler) for 2–3 minutes on each side. Cut the polenta into strips, brush it with melted butter, and barbecue or broil for 1–2 minutes on each side, or until golden. Serve hot with the vegetables.

For a different flavor, use the alternate marinade.

DESSERTS AND SNACKS

Soufflé Pancakes with Strawberries

Makes 4 servings

STRAWBERRIES

16 ounces strawberries, washed, hulled, and halved
3 tablespoons honey
1 tablespoon balsamic vinegar

PANCAKES

8 fluid ounces (1 cup) soy milk
2 eggs, separated
3 teaspoons grated lemon rind
5½ ounces (1 cup) soy or rice flour
1 teaspoon gluten-free baking powder
1 teaspoon vanilla extract
1 tablespoon superfine sugar
Pinch of salt
Powdered sugar for serving

Toss the strawberries with the honey and balsamic vinegar and set aside.

Whisk together the soy milk, egg yolks, lemon rind, flour, baking powder, superfine sugar, vanilla, and salt. In a dry bowl, whisk the egg whites until stiff peaks form. Gently fold the egg whites into the batter until completely blended.

Heat a small amount of the butter in a nonstick frying pan or griddle over medium heat. Pour a large spoonful of batter into the pan and cook for a few minutes on each side, or until golden and puffed. Transfer the pancake to a plate and repeat with the remaining batter.

Serve the strawberries over the warm pancakes. Dust with a little powdered sugar.

Prune and Tofu Whip

Makes 4 servings

4 ounces (½ cup) prunes (preferably unsulfured)
8 ounces (1 cup) tofu
2 tablespoons natural maple syrup or honey

Soak the prunes overnight in water. Drain them, place them in a small saucepan, add water to cover, and simmer for 10–15 minutes, or until really tender. Drain again, reserving the liquid. Place the prunes in a blender and process with the tofu and maple syrup until smooth. Add just enough of the prune cooking liquid to make a thick, soft puree. Pour the mixture into sundae glasses and chill until ready to serve.

Banana Rice

Makes 4 servings

1 pound (2 cups) mashed banana
7 ounces (1 cup) uncooked brown rice
24 fluid ounces (3 cups) soy milk
1 teaspoon pure vanilla extract
Grated zest of 1 lemon
1 teaspoon ground nutmeg

Preheat the oven to 350°F (180°C). Place the banana, rice, soy milk, lemon zest, and vanilla in a 2-quart ovenproof dish and stir well. Bake for 1½–2 hours, or until firm. Sprinkle with nutmeg before serving. Serve the pudding on its own or with stewed fruit.

Banana Smoothie

Makes 4 servings

4 very ripe bananas, peeled and roughly chopped
20 fluid ounces (2½ cups) soy milk, chilled

2 ounces (¼ cup) ground almonds
½ teaspoon ground nutmeg

In a blender, process all ingredients until smooth. Serve chilled.

Mixed Berry Smoothie

Makes 2 servings

16 fluid ounces (2 cups) soy milk
8 ounces (1 cup) natural soy yogurt
1 cup frozen mixed berries, partially thawed
1 banana
1 tablespoon ground almonds

In a blender, process the fruit with the soy milk and yogurt until smooth. Stir in the ground almonds thoroughly. Serve immediately.

Blueberry and Rhubarb Smoothie

Makes 4 servings

1 pound (2 cups) rhubarb, washed, trimmed, and coarsely chopped
1 pound (2 cups) blueberries, washed
32 fluid ounces (4 cups) soy milk, chilled
20 ice cubes, crushed
½ teaspoon vanilla extract
1 teaspoon honey (optional)

In a blender, process all the ingredients until smooth. Serve chilled, with extra ice if desired.

Blueberry and Tofu Brûlée

Makes 4 servings

7 ounces (1 cup) blueberries
9 ounces (1¼ cup) silken tofu
2 tablespoons honey
3 tablespoons soft brown sugar

Preheat the broiler. In a blender, process the blueberries, tofu, and honey until smooth. Pour the mixture into 4 ovenproof ramekins. Sprinkle the sugar on top and broil for a few minutes, until the sugar forms a hard, golden layer.

Dried Fruit Compote

Makes 4 servings

8 ounces mixed dried, unsulfured fruits, such as peaches, prunes,
    apples, apricots, and pears
5 fluid ounces orange juice
4 whole cloves
Four 1-inch sticks cinnamon
Juice and zest of 1 lemon

The day before serving, wash the fruit and place it in a bowl with the orange juice, spices, lemon juice, and zest. Soak overnight. Next day, if all the juice has been absorbed, add 2 tablespoons water. Place the mixture in a saucepan, bring it to the boil, then cover and simmer on a very low heat for 10–15 minutes.

Transfer to a serving bowl, removing the cinnamon and cloves. Serve warm or at room temperature, topped with soy yogurt.

Fresh Fruit Salad

Makes 4 servings

1 apple, peeled and sliced
1 banana, peeled and sliced
Juice of 4 lemons
1 orange, peeled and segmented
1 grapefruit, peeled and segmented
4 ounces seedless grapes, halved
2 kiwifruit, peeled and sliced
2 teaspoons orange juice
4 sprigs of mint

Toss the apple and banana in the lemon juice. This will prevent discoloration. Combine all fruits in a serving bowl and add the orange juice. Serve chilled and decorated with sprigs of mint.

Banana and Tofu Cream

Makes 4 servings

7 ounces firm tofu
7 ounces banana
3 ounces ground almonds
Pinch of cinnamon
2 teaspoons sliced almonds

In a blender, process the tofu and banana together until creamy. If necessary, sieve the mixture. Add the ground almonds and mix well. Spoon into 4 bowls and sprinkle with the cinnamon and a few sliced almonds.

Passion Fruit Fool

Makes 4 servings

6 ripe passion fruit
5 fluid ounces soy milk
3 teaspoons cornstarch
2 tablespoons water
4 fluid ounces (½ cup) soy yogurt
1 tablespoon clear honey

Halve the passion fruit and scoop the pulp into a bowl. Gently heat the soy milk. Blend the cornstarch and water into a smooth paste and then stir into the hot milk. Over low heat, stir until the mixture has thickened. Add the yogurt and honey, stir thoroughly, and allow the mixture to cool. Combine the sauce and the passion fruit pulp, and then spoon the mixture into serving dishes. Chill the dishes for 3–4 minutes before serving.

Rhubarb and Ginger Mousse

Makes 4 servings

16 ounces rhubarb
Grated rind and juice of ½ orange
3 tablespoons clear honey
2 tablespoons water
¼ teaspoon ground ginger
2 teaspoons powdered gelatin (or vegetarian alternative)
2 egg whites

Trim the rhubarb and chop into 1-inch pieces. Place it in a pan with the honey, orange juice, orange rind, and ginger, and simmer gently until the fruit is soft. In a small bowl set in a pan of hot water, dissolve the gelatin in 2 tablespoons of water. Stir until the mixture is completely clear. Add the gelatin to the rhubarb and beat until thoroughly combined.

Cool the rhubarb mixture until it is half-set. Whisk the egg whites until stiff and fold them lightly into the mixture. Spoon it into decorative glasses and chill until completely set.

Phyto Fix Bars

Makes 16 bars

2 ounces (¼ cup) sesame seeds
4 ounces (½ cup) golden flaxseeds
2 ounces (¼ cup) sunflower seeds
2 ounces (¼ cup) pumpkin seeds
4 ounces (½ cup) raisins, golden raisins, or currants
2 ounces (¼ cup) dried unsulfured apricots, chopped
3 ounces (¾ cup) soy protein powder
4 ounces (4 cups) puffed rice
2 teaspoons mixed spice
2 teaspoons powdered ginger (optional)
4 fluid ounces (½ cup) date syrup
2 fluid ounces (¼ cup) ginger or rice syrup
10 fluid ounces (1¼ cup) soy milk

Preheat the oven to 350°F (180°C). Combine the dry ingredients and fruits in a bowl. Add the syrups and milk and mix thoroughly. Grease 12 × 8-inch baking pan. Pour in the mixture and smooth the surface. Bake for 20 minutes until golden brown. Allow to cool, then cut into 16 bars.

Fruit Bars

Makes 12 bars

4 ounces (½ cups) dried unsulfured apricots, diced
1 teaspoon grated orange rind
4 fluid ounces (½ cup) orange juice
2 ounces (¼ cup) almonds, chopped
2 ounces (¼ cup) shredded coconut
2 ounces (2 cups) puffed rice
4 ounces (½ cup) ground almonds
2 ounces (¼ cup) dried fruit, such as raisins, apples, and peaches
Extra shredded coconut for baking

Preheat the oven to 350°F. Simmer the apricots and orange rind in the orange juice for 5 minutes, or until soft. Toast the chopped almonds and the coconut in the oven for about 10 minutes, making sure they don't burn. In a blender, process the apricot mixture, coconut, puffed rice, and ground almonds. (This mixture is quite sticky, so stop the blender and scrape it from the sides once or twice.)

Pour the mixture into a bowl and add the chopped toasted almonds and additional dried fruit. Mix by hand into a large ball. Line a baking sheet with foil and sprinkle it with extra coconut. Flatten the mixture onto the baking sheet and sprinkle with more coconut. Cut into bars and allow to dry (preferably overnight) before storing in a sealed container. Use within 1 week.

Chapter 13

DIETARY RESOURCES

Phyto-Rich and Gluten-Free Products

It can be difficult to identify ready-made foods that are rich in phytoestrogens as well as being gluten-free, and not laden with sugar or additives. These are some brands and varieties I recommend that are widely available in the US. For recommended brands and varieties available in the UK, please see Appendix 1 (p. 229).

Crackers

Top Picks

Flackers Organic Flaxseed Crackers
Go Raw Flax Snax
Le Pains de Fleurs Crispbread
Lundberg Rice Cakes

Crackers Containing Unprocessed Seed Oils

Kashi Teff Thins — a variety of crackers made with alternative grains
Mary's Gone Crackers — a selection of tasty, thin crackers
Simple Mills — a good variety of almond-flour products, including crackers
    and waffles

Crackers with Phytoestrogens

Mary's Gone Crackers — gluten-free, organic

Breads

Top Picks

These are all gluten-free, using a variety of nutritious grains.

Amy's Organic Sandwich Rounds — made with organic rice flour
Canyon Bakehouse — all whole-grain products
Food for Life Sprouted for Life — made with quinoa, millet, and chia seeds

Breads Containing Unprocessed Seed Oils

Trader Joe's Gluten-Free Multigrain Bread — with brown rice, sorghum, teff, and amaranth

Other Bread Options

The following brands of bread are more highly processed than those listed above but are also more widely available.

Rudi's Gluten-Free Bakery Multigrain and Home-Style Breads
Udi's Gluten-Free Omega Flax and Fiber Bread and Sprouted Grains Artisan Bread

Pasta

Andean Dream Quinoa and Rice Pasta
DeBoles Rice Pasta
Eden Mung Bean Pasta
Explore Cuisine Black Bean Pasta
Jovial Organic Whole Grain Rice Pasta
Tinkyada Brown Rice Pasta

Low-Calorie Pasta Substitutes

Gold Mine Kelp Noodles
House Foods Traditional Shirataki Yam Noodles
Riced cauliflower (sold frozen)
Sea Tangle Kelp Noodles
Spiralized zucchini and summer squash (homemade or store-bought precut)

Cookies

Top Picks

These brands are all healthier choices for snacks, without added sugar. Some varieties include sprouted seeds and omega-3-rich nuts.

Caveman Cookies
Chunkie Dunkies
Coco-Roons
Enjoy Life Crunch Handcrafted
Go Raw Sprouted Cookies
Hail Merry Macaroons
Mary's Gone Crackers Cookies
Simple Mills

Cookies Containing Unprocessed Seed Oils

Aldi's Live G-Free Soft Baked Cookies
Enjoy Life Soft Baked Cookies
Lucy's Cookies
Pamela's Simple Bites
Trader Joe's Soft-Baked Snickerdoodles

Flours

Arrowhead Mills all-purpose and individual gluten-free grain flours
Bob's Red Mill all-purpose and individual gluten-free grain flours

Baking Mixes

Arrowhead Mills Organic Gluten-Free Pancake and Baking Mix
Birch Benders Paleo Pancakes
Enjoy Life Muffin Mixes
Namaste Foods Waffle and Pancake Mix
Simple Mills bread and muffin mixes

Cold Cereals

I usually discourage consumption of cold cereals because they are notoriously high in sugar — more of a dessert than a breakfast. However, these options are either sugar-free or low in sugar.

Arrowhead Mills (Organic Rice Flakes, Organic Corn Flakes, Organic Maple
    Buckwheat Flakes)
Back to Nature Sprout & Shine
Erewhon Crispy Brown Rice Cereal
Nature's Path Organic Whole O's

Hot Cereals

Ancient Harvest Quinoa Flakes
Arrowhead Mills (Rice & Shine, Quinoa & Oat, Organic Corn Grits, Quinoa
    Rice & Shine)
Bob's Red Mill Gluten-Free Oats
Glutenfreeda Instant Oatmeal
Pocono Cream of Buckwheat

Gluten-Free Treats

Daiya frozen cheesecake
Hail Merry baked goods
Kashi Gluten-Free Waffles
Luna & Larry's coconut milk ice creams
So Delicious coconut, almond, and cashew milk ice creams

Soy Products

Beware of soy products containing monosodium glutamate (MSG), the food additive E621, as some people can be sensitive to it and find it causes anything from headaches to thermal surges which resemble hot flashes, shortness of breath, or rapid heartbeats. On product labels, this additive can be hidden under other names such as yeast extract, hydrolyzed yeast, and autolyzed yeast. Any soy-based savory foods with additional flavoring may contain MSG. The following foods do not contain MSG.

Amy's Frozen Meals (choose those with tofu)
Cascadian Farms Organic Shelled Edamame
Explore Cuisine Organic Edamame Spaghetti
LiteLife Organic Tempeh (various flavors)
Miso Master Organic Miso
Nasoya Organic Tofu
Plant Pure Frozen Meals (choose those with tofu)
So Delicious Organic Soy Milk Ice Cream
Stonyfield Organic Dairy-Free Yogurt
West Soy Organic Tempeh
Wildwood Organic Sprouted Tofu (and marinated tofu)

Caffeine-Free Teas

Bigelow caffeine-free herbal teas
Celestial Seasonings caffeine-free fruit teas
Numi assorted caffeine-free herbal teas (Rooibos Chai, Mint, Chamomile
    Lemon, Turmeric Three Roots)

Tazo assorted caffeine-free herbal teas (Calm, Mint, Passion, Organic Baked
   Cinnamon Apple, Sweet Cinnamon Spice)
Trader Joe's Herbal Tea, Ginger Turmeric
Trader Joe's Pumpkin Spice Rooibos Herbal Blend Tea
Twinings of London Rooibos
Yogi assorted caffeine-free herbal teas (Bedtime, Immune Support, Cold Season,
   Throat Comfort, Stress Relief, Stomach Ease, Relax Mind)

Nutritional Content of Foods

These lists show the foods that contain the highest quantity of each nutrient by weight.
(Note that standard serving sizes may differ considerably from the specified weight.)
Unless otherwise stated, foods listed are raw.

Vitamin A

Micrograms per 100 grams (3.5 ounces)

Lamb liver	15,000
Butter	815
Margarine	800
Cheese, cheddar	325
Hot cereal, made with milk	56
Milk, whole	52
Herring, grilled	49
Milk	21

Vitamin B1 (thiamine)

Milligrams per 100 grams (3.5 ounces)

Wheat germ	2.01
Brazil nuts	1.00
Cornflakes	1.00
Rice Krispies	1.00
Flour, whole wheat	0.47
Walnuts	0.40

Bacon, cooked	0.35
Flour, all-purpose white	0.30
Plaice, steamed	0.30
Almonds	0.24
Spaghetti, cooked	0.21
Salmon, steamed	0.20
Corn (kernels cut off the cob)	0.20
Lentils, boiled	0.14
Soybeans, boiled	0.12
Red bell pepper	0.12
Potatoes, new, boiled	0.11
Savoy cabbage, boiled	0.10

Vitamin B2 (riboflavin)

Milligrams per 100 grams (3.5 ounces)

Cornflakes	1.50
Rice Krispies	1.50
Almonds	0.75
Cheese, cheddar	0.40

Lamb leg, cooked	0.38	Cod, grilled	1.70
Egg, boiled	0.35	Bread, white	1.70
Beef, topside, cooked	0.35	Flour, all-purpose white	1.50
Shrimp, boiled	0.34	Rice, brown	1.30
Flour, soy	0.31	Cabbage, boiled	0.30
Cheese, cottage	0.26	Apple	0.20
Turkey, roasted	0.21	Cheese, cottage	0.13
Chicken, roasted	0.19	Milk, low-fat or skim	0.09
Avocado	0.18	Milk, whole	0.08
Herring, grilled	0.18	Egg, boiled	0.07
Milk, low-fat	0.18	Cheese, cheddar	0.07
Milk, whole	0.17		
Red bell pepper	0.15		
Salmon, baked	0.11		
Peanuts	0.10		

Vitamin B6 (pyridoxine)

Milligrams per 100 grams (3.5 ounces)

Special K	2.20
Cornflakes	1.80
Rice Krispies	1.80
Muesli	1.60
Walnuts	0.67
Hazelnuts	0.59
Peanuts	0.59
Salmon, baked	0.57
Flour, soy	0.57
Cod, grilled	0.38
Avocado	0.36
Turkey, roasted	0.33
Herring, grilled	0.33
Beef, topside, cooked	0.33
Potatoes, boiled	0.32
Brazil nuts	0.31
Banana	0.29
Lentils, boiled	0.28
Chicken, roasted	0.26
Grapefruit juice	0.23

Vitamin B3 (niacin)

Milligrams per 100 grams (3.5 ounces)

Cornflakes	16.00
Rice Krispies	16.00
Peanuts	13.80
Shrimp, boiled	9.50
Turkey, roasted	8.50
Chicken, roasted	8.20
Salmon, baked	7.00
Lamb leg, cooked	6.60
Muesli	6.50
Beef, topside, cooked	6.50
Flour, whole wheat	5.70
Bread, whole wheat	4.10
Herring, grilled	4.00
Almonds	3.10
Red bell pepper	2.20
Flour, soy	2.00

Vitamin B12 (cyanocobalamine)

Micrograms per 100 grams (3.5 ounces)

Sardines, in oil	28.0
Nori seaweed	27.5
Oysters, raw	15.0
Mackerel, fried	10.
Herring, cooked	6.0
Herring roe, fried	6.0
Salmon, steamed	6.0
Grape Nuts	5.0
Tuna, in oil	5.0
Duck, cooked	3.0
Turkey, dark meat	3.0
Squid, frozen	2.9
Taramasalata	2.9
Kombu seaweed	2.8
Eggs, whole, free-range	2.7
Cheese, Edam	2.1
Beef, lean	2.0

Folate (Folic Acid)

Micrograms per 100 grams (3.5 ounces)

Calf liver, fried	320
Cornflakes	250
Rice Krispies	250
Lamb liver, fried	240
Chickpeas	180
Asparagus	155
Sweet corn, boiled (kernels off the cob)	150
Brussels sprouts	110
Peanuts	110

Spinach, boiled	90
Hazelnuts	72
Artichoke	68
Walnuts	66
Broccoli	64
Green beans, boiled	57
Cauliflower	51
Almonds	48
Parsnips, boiled	48
Peas, frozen	47

Vitamin C

Milligrams per 100 grams (3.5 ounces)

Black currants	115
Strawberries	77
Brussels sprouts	60
Kiwifruit	59
Orange	54
Apple juice	49
Lychees, fresh	45
Broccoli	44
Kumquats	39
Mango	37
Nectarine	37
Grapefruit	36
Bran flakes	35
Raspberries	32
Peach	31
Cauliflower	27
Satsuma	27
Melon, cantaloupe	26
Cabbage, boiled	20

Vitamin D

*Micrograms per 100 grams (3.5 ounces)
except where noted*

Sockeye salmon (canned)	17.9
Rainbow trout, farmed and cooked	16.2
Mackerel, Pacific and Jack, cooked	9.7
Margarine	8.00
Halibut, Atlantic and Pacific, cooked	4.7
Kellogg's Start	4.20
Cornflakes	2.80
Rice Krispies	2.80
Mushrooms, morel, raw	1.7
Egg, boiled	1.1
Cheese, cheddar	0.26
Cheese, fromage frais	0.05
Milk, 1 cup of 1% or 2%	2.9
Soy milk, 1 cup	2.9
Almond milk, 1 cup	2.4

Vitamin E

Milligrams per 100 grams (3.5 ounces)

Sunflower oil	49
Hazelnuts	25
Almonds	24
Rapeseed oil	18
Pine nuts	14
Peanuts	10
Brazil nuts	7
Sweet potato, baked	6
Olive oil	5
Peanut butter	5
Walnuts	4
Avocado	3
Mushrooms, fried	3
Onions, raw, dried	3
Butter	2
Olives	2
Spinach, boiled	2
Parsley	2
Watercress	1

Calcium

Milligrams per 100 grams (3.5 ounces)

Parmesan	1220
Sesame seeds	1160
Cheese, cheddar	720
Sardines, canned	766
Flour, all-purpose white	450
Dried figs	280
Almonds	240
Soy flour	210
Yogurt, low-fat	190
Shrimp, boiled	150
Spinach, boiled	150
Milk, 2% fat	120
Soybeans, boiled	83
Cheese, cottage	73
Brazil nuts	700
Peanuts	60
Egg, boiled	57

Chromium

Micrograms per 100 grams (3.5 ounces)

Egg yolk	183
Molasses	121
Brewer's yeast	117
Beef	570
Cheese, hard	56
Liver, fried	55
Fruit juice, fresh	47

Iron

Milligrams per 100 grams (3.5 ounces)

Liver, fried	10
Mussels, boiled	6.0
Flour, soy	6.9
Cornflakes	6.7
Rice Krispies	6.7
Muesli	5.6
Oysters, raw	5.0
Flour, whole wheat	3.9
Lentils, boiled	3.5
Almonds	3.0
Sardines, canned	3.0
Soybeans, boiled	3.0
Beef, topside, cooked	2.8
Lamb leg, cooked	2.7
Bread, whole wheat	2.7
Brazil nuts	2.5
Peanuts	2.5
Flour, all-purpose white	2.0
Egg, boiled	1.9
Spinach, boiled	1.7
Bread, white	1.6

Baked beans	1.4
Spaghetti, whole wheat, cooked	1.4
Green bell pepper	1.2

Magnesium

Milligrams per 100 grams (3.5 ounces)

Brazil nuts	410
Almonds	270
Flour, soy	240
Peanuts	210
Flour, whole wheat	120
Muesli	85
Bread, whole wheat	76
Soybeans, boiled	63
Rice, brown, boiled	43
Shrimp, boiled	42
Spaghetti, whole wheat	42
Banana	34
Lentils, boiled	34
Herring, grilled	32
Baked beans	31
Spinach, boiled	31
Salmon, baked	29
Lamb leg, cooked	28
Turkey, roasted	27
Cod, grilled	26

Selenium

Micrograms per 100 grams (3.5 ounces)

Brazil nuts	1,900
Flour, whole wheat	53
Lentils, boiled	40

Bread, whole wheat	35
Bread, white	28
Cheese, cheddar	12
Egg, boiled	11
Soybeans, boiled	5
Almonds	4
Cheese, cottage	4
Rice, white	4
Flour, all-purpose white	4
Peanuts	3
Baked beans	2
Cornflakes	2
Orange	2
Milk, whole, low-fat, or skim	1

Zinc

Milligrams per 100 g (3.5 ounces)

Beef, topside, cooked	5.5
Lamb leg, cooked	5.3
Brazil nuts	4.2
Peanuts	3.5
Almonds	3.2
Flour, whole wheat	2.9
Muesli	2.5
Turkey, roasted	2.4
Cheese, cheddar	2.3
Bread, whole wheat	1.8
Shrimp, boiled	1.6
Chicken, roasted	1.5
Lentils, boiled	1.4
Egg, boiled	1.3
Spaghetti, whole wheat, cooked	1.1
Soybeans, boiled	0.9
Rice, brown	0.7
Rice, white	0.7
Cheese, cottage	0.6
Spinach, boiled	0.6
Bread, white	0.6
Flour, all-purpose white	0.6

Essential Fatty Acids

Amounts of these fats are hard to quantify precisely. Good sources for the two families of essential fatty acids are listed below.

Omega-6
Sunflower oil
Rapeseed oil
Corn oil
Almonds
Walnuts
Brazil nuts
Sunflower seeds
Soy products, including tofu

Omega-3
Oily fish (mackerel, herring, salmon, trout)
Walnuts
Walnut oil
Rapeseed oil
Olive oil

Appendix I

UK FOOD RECOMMENDATIONS

Recommended Products and Brands

The products and brands listed here can be found at Holland & Barrett, Tesco, Waitrose, or www.planetorganic.com.

Bread

Burgen Gluten-Free Soya and Linseed Bread
Genius Gluten-Free Bread

Cereal

Nature's Path Organic Gluten-Free Mesa Sunrise
Puffed rice cereal

Crackers

RAW Vibrant Living Flax Pumpkin Crackers
Rude Health Buckwheat & Chia Crackers

Soya Products

Alpro Natural (Plain) Soya Yogurt
Alpro Simply Vanilla Desserts
Sojade So Soja yogurt alternatives

Provamel Organic Soya Drink (Unsweetened)
Provamel Yogurts

Snack Bars

Deliciously Ella Almond & Blueberry Energy Ball
Deliciously Ella Cashew & Ginger Energy Ball
Nakd Blueberry Muffin Fruit and Nut Bars
Nakd Berry Delight Fruit and Nut Bars
Trek Blueberry and Pumpkin Protein Nut Bar

Prepared Food Recommendations for Eating on the Run

Menus vary depending on the season. The following are examples of what to look for.

Available at Pret a Manger

Bircher Muesli (with Gluten-Free Granola)
Butternut and Lentil Dhal Soup
Salmon and Mango Salad Bowl
Tamari and Ginger Chicken Salad Bowl
Smashed Avocado on Gluten-Free Bread Sandwich
Sweet Potato Falafel & Smashed Beets Veggie Box

Available at Starbucks

Chicken and Avocado Protein Bowl
Vegan Roasted Vegetable Salad

Appendix II

FORMS AND WEBSITES

Provided here are the Natural Menopause Solution worksheet and diaries for recording your daily diet and assessing and tracking your symptoms. Don't underestimate their value. The success of my program is directly related to the degree to which women follow it.

As you progress through the six-week program, use the natural menopause solution worksheet (p. 232), diet diary (p. 235), and menopause symptom diary (p. 241) to record how you are feeling, the choices you are making in order to feel better, and the changes you notice.

Using the worksheet, take a little time to identify your main symptoms, how they impinge on your life, and how you would like to feel. You'll find this information useful to refer back to.

Complete the diet diary daily during the six-week program, listing all foods, drinks, and supplements consumed. Keeping accurate records of your diet, activity level, and well-being encourages you to stick with the program; helps identify foods, environmental factors, and habits that may aggravate symptoms; and documents your progress.

Women with mild to moderate menopause symptoms can very often manage with self-help measures, while those experiencing more severe, debilitating symptoms may need additional help and support. If you suffer from brain fog, insomnia, and anxiety, for example, it may too much for you to manage alone.

If you would like some personal help or would like to join a virtual Six-Week Natural Menopause Solution class or a live question-and-answer session, please follow the links to my website on page 244. My team and I also provide a three-month coaching course to build on the Six-Week Natural Menopause Solution. You are most welcome to join us.

Good luck with your journey!

NATURAL MENOPAUSE
SOLUTION WORKSHEET

Date:

My worst symptoms are:

How these symptoms affect my life:

How these symptoms affect my self-esteem:

How these symptoms affect my relationships with my partner, family, and friends:

How these symptoms affect my work life and productivity:

How I'm feeling today:

How I would like to feel and be:

What I believe is preventing me from feeling well:

How urgent it is to me to overcome these symptoms:

1　　**2**　　**3**　　**4**　　**5**　　**6**　　**7**　　**8**　　**9**　　**10**

Not urgent　　　　　　　　　　　　　　　　　　　　　　Very urgent

How willing I am to make diet and lifestyle changes:

1　　**2**　　**3**　　**4**　　**5**　　**6**　　**7**　　**8**　　**9**　　**10**

Not very willing　　　　　　　　　　　　　Willing to do whatever it takes

Self-Assessment

In the table below, record your results from the self-assessment quizzes in chapters 1–6 when you start the program and at the end of week 6. Compare the before and after scores to see the progress you've made.

	Start of Week 1	End of Week 6
Assess your symptoms (Chapter 1)		
Do you suffer from food sensitivities? (Chapter 2)		
Do food and drink cravings have a hold over you? (Chapter 2)		
How fit are you? (Chapter 4)		
How's your libido? (Chapter 5)		
How stressed are you? (Chapter 5)		
How sharp is your brain? (Chapter 6)		
How's your self-esteem? (Chapter 6)		
What's your risk of heart disease? (Chapter 9)		
How strong are your bones? (Chapter 10)		

Natural Menopause Solution Worksheet (*continued*)

Current weight: ___pounds or ___kilograms

Ideal weight: ___pounds or ___kilograms

Possible nutritional deficiencies (see chapter 2):

Dietary changes that may help me (see chapter 2):

Supplements that may help me:

My relaxation plan:

My exercise plan:

Notes

DIET DIARY
WEEK 1

	Breakfast	Lunch	Dinner	Snacks	Other Notes (exercise, symptoms, supplements)
Day 1					
Day 2					
Day 3					
Day 4					
Day 5					
Day 6					
Day 7					

DIET DIARY
WEEK 2

	Breakfast	Lunch	Dinner	Snacks	Other Notes (exercise, symptoms, supplements)
Day 1					
Day 2					
Day 3					
Day 4					
Day 5					
Day 6					
Day 7					

DIET DIARY
WEEK 3

	Breakfast	Lunch	Dinner	Snacks	Other Notes (exercise, symptoms, supplements)
Day 1					
Day 2					
Day 3					
Day 4					
Day 5					
Day 6					
Day 7					

DIET DIARY
WEEK 4

	Breakfast	Lunch	Dinner	Snacks	Other Notes (exercise, symptoms, supplements)
Day 1					
Day 2					
Day 3					
Day 4					
Day 5					
Day 6					
Day 7					

DIET DIARY
WEEK 5

	Breakfast	Lunch	Dinner	Snacks	Other Notes (exercise, symptoms, supplements)
Day 1					
Day 2					
Day 3					
Day 4					
Day 5					
Day 6					
Day 7					

DIET DIARY
WEEK 6

	Breakfast	Lunch	Dinner	Snacks	Other Notes (exercise, symptoms, supplements)
Day 1					
Day 2					
Day 3					
Day 4					
Day 5					
Day 6					
Day 7					

MENOPAUSE SYMPTOM DIARY

Grading of Symptoms

0   None (or you can leave these columns blank)

1   Mild: present but does not interfere with activities

2   Moderate: present and interferes with activities, but not disabling

3   Severe: disabling

Symptom	WEEK					
	1	2	3	4	5	6
Hot flashes						
Facial or body flushing						
Excessive perspiration						
Night sweats						
Palpitations						
Panic attacks						
Generalized aches and pains						
Depression						
Numbness or tingling in arms or legs						
Headaches						
Backache						
Fatigue/lack of vitality						
Confusion						
Forgetfulness						

Menopause Symptom Diary (*continued*)

Symptom	WEEK					
	1	**2**	**3**	**4**	**5**	**6**
Difficulty concentrating						
Irritability						
Anxiety						
Nervousness						
Loss of confidence						
Insomnia						
Giddiness or dizziness						
Pain or difficulty with urination						
Frequent urination						
Stress incontinence						
Constipation						
Abdominal bloating						
Diarrhea, gas						
Itchy vagina						
Dry vagina						
Painful intercourse						
Decreased sex drive						
Water retention						

Additional Data	WEEK					
	1	2	3	4	5	6
Weight in pounds or kilograms measured on the same day and time each week)						
Menstrual period and related symptoms (if applicable)						
Frequency of sexual intercourse (note days)						
Enjoyment of sexual intercourse (on a scale of 0 to 10)						

Notes

USEFUL WEBSITES

Maryon Stewart's website: maryonstewart.com
- USA Six-Week Natural Menopause Solution: maryonstewart.com/six-week-us
- UK Six-Week Natural Menopause Solution:
- maryonstewart.com/six-week
- Online shop for recommended books and supplements: maryonstewart.com/shop

Corporate courses: maryonstewart.com/healthywiseandwell

National Association of Cognitive-Behavioral Therapists: www.nacbt.org

National Osteoporosis Foundation: www.nof.org
- National Osteoporosis Foundation bone health calculator: www.iofbonehealth.org/calcium-calculator

North American Menopause Society: www.menopause.com

Sleep Association: www.sleepassociation.org

ACKNOWLEDGMENTS

This book wouldn't have been possible if it weren't for the many women who have trusted me enough to put their well-being in my hands over the last twenty-seven years.

My thanks are also due to the researchers around the world whose work has made it possible to for me to put together a scientifically based, nondrug program. I'm particularly grateful to Mark Messina for his extensive research on naturally occurring estrogen; to Alan Stewart, Stephen Davies, and Leo Galland for their pioneering work in nutrition; and to Dr. Emmanuela Wolloch for writing the foreword to my first American book.

I am enormously grateful to Julie Whittaker and Barbara Hendricks for working so hard behind the scenes to create my website and support network, and to my extended team who are on the mission with me to change the paradigm of menopause so that instead of dreading it, women can welcome it as a time to focus on themselves for their "midlife refuel." Gratitude also goes to Jane Garton for her editing skills, Suzie Sawyer for helping refine our course content, Staci Shacter for her contribution to the US food lists, and Dr. Susan Aldridge for helping with the literature searches and getting the medical references in order. Last, but by no means least, my gratitude and love to my wonderful husband Ben, who not only meticulously proofread my work but also fed and nurtured me, allowing me to focus on my passion to help women around the world to reclaim their well-being at midlife.

My deepest gratitude to you all.

MEDICAL REFERENCES

General References

American Medical Association. *Essential guide to menopause*. New York: Pocket Books, 2004

Bruinsma K, Taren DL. Chocolate: food or drug? *Journal of the American Dietetic Association*. 1999: 99(10): 1249–1256

Berg G, Hammar M (eds). *The modern management of the menopause*. New York, London: Parthenon, 1994

Dennerstein L, Wood C, Westmore A. *Hysterectomy: new options and advances*, 2nd edn. Melbourne, Oxford: Oxford University Press, 1995

Peacock K, Ketvertis K. Menopause NCBI Bookshelf StatPearls. Treasure Island, FL: StatPearls Publishing, 2020

Pizzorno JE, Murray MT (eds). *Textbook of natural medicine*. Edinburgh: Churchill Livingstone, 1999

Souhami RL, Moxham J (eds). *Textbook of medicine*, 4th edn. Edinburgh: Churchill Livingstone, 2002

Steinke D. *Flash Count Diary: a new story about the menopause*. New York: Sarah Crichton Books / Farrar, Straus and Giroux, 2019

Stewart M. *Cruising through the menopause*. London: Vermilion, 2000

Stewart M. *The phyto factor*. London: Vermilion, 2000

Stewart M, Stewart A. *The natural health bible: an A–Z guide to drug-free health*. Sydney: New Holland, 2002

Werbach MR. *Textbook of nutritional medicine*. Tarzana, CA: Third Line Press, 1999

Prevalence and Surveys

Anderson DJ, Chung HF, Seib CA, et al. Obesity, smoking and risk of vasomotor menopausal symptoms: a pooled analysis of eight cohort studies. *American Journal of Obstetrics and Gynecology* 2019; Am J Obstet Gynecol. 2020; 222(5): 478.e1-478.e17. doi:10.1016/j.ajog.2019.10.103

Avis NE, Crawford SL, Greendale G, et al. Duration of menopausal vasomotor symptoms over the menopause transition. *JAMA Internal Medicine* 2015; 175(4): 531–539

Converso D, Viotti S, Sottimano I, et al. The relationship between menopausal symptoms and burnout: a cross-sectional study among nurses. *BMC Women's Health* 2019; 19(1): 148

Creedy DK, Sidebotham M, Gamble J, et al. Prevalence of burnout, depression, anxiety and stress in Australian midwives: a cross-sectional survey. *BMC Pregnancy and Childbirth* 2017; 17(1): 13

Dias RCA, Kulak J Jr, Ferreira da Costa EH, et al. Fibromyalgia, sleep disturbance and menopause: is there a relationship? A literature review. *International Journal of Rheumatic Diseases* 2019; 22(11): 1961–1971

Gartoulla P, Bell RJ, Worsley R, et al. Moderate–severely bothersome vasomotor symptoms are associated with lowered psychological general wellbeing in women at midlife. *Maturitas* 2015; 81(4): 487–492

Gartoulla PI, Worsley R, Bell RJ, et al. Moderate to severe vasomotor and sexual symptoms remain problematic for women aged 60 to 65 years. *Menopause* 2015; 22(7): 694–701

Hgai FW. Relationships between menopausal symptoms, sense of coherence, coping strategies, and quality of life. *Menopause* 2019; 26(7): 758–764

Klino JM, Kelly M, Rullo J, et al. Association between menopausal symptoms and relationship distress. *Maturitas* 2019; 130: 1–5

Larroy C, Marin Martin C, Lopez-Picado A, et al. The impact of perimenopausal symptomatology, sociodemographic status and knowledge of menopause of women's quality of life. *Archives of Gynecology and Obstetrics* 2020 Apr; 301(4): 1061–1068

Loehr A. How menopause silently affects 27 million women at work every day. https://www.fastcompany.com/3056703/how-menopause-silently-affects-27-million-women-at-work-every-day. Fast Company: How Menopause Silently Affects 27 Million Women at Work Every Day, February 17, 2016

Minkin MJ, Reiter S, Maamari R. Prevalence of postmenopausal symptoms in North America and Europe. *Menopause* 2015; 22(11): 1231–1238

Namazi N, Sadeghi R, Behboodi Moghadam Z. Social determinants of health in menopause: an integrative review. *International Journal of Women's Health* 2019; 11: 637–647

Nappi RE, Palacios S, Panay N, et al. Vulvar and vaginal atrophy in four European countries: evidence from the European REVIVE survey. *Climacteric* 2016; 19(2): 188–197

Peng K, Yao P, Kartsonaki C, et al. Menopause and risk of hip fracture in middle-aged Chinese women: a 10-year follow-up of China Kadoorie Biobank. *Menopause* 2020 Mar; 27(3): 311–318

Prairie BA, Wisnirewski SR, Luther J, et al. Symptoms of depressed mood, disturbed sleep, and sexual problems in midlife women: cross-sectional data from the Study of Women's Health Across the Nation. *Journal of Women's Health* 2015; 24(2): 119–126

Süss H, Ehlert U. Psychological resilience during the perimenopause. *Maturitas* 2020; 131: 48–56

Zolfaghari S, Yao C, Thompson C, et al. Effects of menopause on sleep quality and sleep disorders: Canadian Longitudinal Study on Aging. *Menopause* 2020 Mar; 27(3): 295–304

Menopause and Hormone Therapy

Alperin M, Burnett L, Lukacz E, et al. The mysteries of menopause: health, clinical and scientific gaps. *Menopause* 2019; 28(1): 103–111

Anderson GL, Limacher M, Assaf AR, et al. Effects of conjugated equine estrogen in postmenopausal women with hysterectomy: the Women's Health Initiative randomized controlled trial. *JAMA* 2004; 291(14): 1701–1712

Bansai R, Aggarwal N. Menopausal hot flashes: a review. *Journal of Midlife Health.* 2019; 10(1): 6–13

Beral V, et al. Breast cancer and hormone replacement therapy in the Million Women Study. *Lancet* 2003; 362(9382): 419–427

Botteri E, Støer NC, Weiderpass E, et al. Menopausal hormone therapy and risk of melanoma: a nationwide register-based study in Finland. *Cancer Epidemiology, Biomarkers and Prevention* 2019; 28(11): 1857–1860

Burkard T, Rauch M, Spoendin J, et al. Risk of hand osteoarthritis in new users of hormone replacement therapy: A nested case-control analysis. *Maturitas* 2020; 2020 Feb; 132: 17–23

Cohen JL. Evaluation of efficacy of a skin care regimen containing methyl estradiolpropanoate (MEP) for treating estrogen deficient skin. *Journal of Drugs in Dermatology* 2019; 18(12): 1226–1230

Collaborative Group on Hormonal Factors in Breast Cancer. Type and timing of menopausal hormone therapy and breast cancer risk: individual participant meta-analysis of the worldwide epidemiological evidence. *Lancet* Published online 2019 Sep 28; 394(10204): 1159–1168

Comhaire FH, Depypere HT. Hormones, herbal preparations and nutriceuticals for a better life after the menopause, part 1. 2015. *Climacteric* 18(3): 364–371

Davies M, Hameda H. Hormone replacement therapy: changes in prescribing practice. *BMJ* 2019; 364: l633

DeNeui T, Berg J, Howson A. Best practices in care for menopausal patients: 15 years after the Women's Health Initiative. *Journal of the American Association of Nurse Practitioners* 2019; 31(7): 420–427

Dotlic J, Nicevic S, Kurtajic I, et al. Hormonal therapy in menopausal transition: implications for improvement of health-related quality of life. *Gynecological Endocrinology* 2020 Apr; 36(4): 327–332

Fait T. Menopause hormone therapy: latest developments and clinical practice. *Drugs Context.* 2019; Jan 2: 8: 212551

Gambacciani M, Cagnacci A, Lello S. Hormone replacement therapy and prevention of chronic conditions. *Climacteric* 2019; 22(3): 303–306

Gass ML, Stuenkel CA, Utian WH, et al. Use of compounded hormone therapy in the United States: report of the North American Menopause Society Survey. *Menopause* 2015; 22(12): 1276–1285

Geiger PJ, Eisenlohr-Moul T, Gordon JL, et al. Effects of perimenopausal transdermal estradiol on self-reported sleep, independent of its effect on vasomotor system bother and depressive symptoms. *Menopause* 2019; 26(11): 1318–1323

Hale GE, Hughes CL, Robboy SJ, et al. A double-blind randomized study on the effects of red clover isoflavones on the endometrium. *Menopause* 2001; 8(5): 338–346

Hawkes N. HRT increases risk of blood clots and stroke, finds new analysis. *BMJ* 2015; 350: h1336

Hsieh E, Nunez-Smith M, Henrich JB. Needs and priorities in women's health training: perspectives from an internal medicine residency program. *Journal of Women's Health* 2013; 22(8): 667–672

Jack G, Riach K, Bariolo E, et al. Menopause in the workplace: what employers should be doing. *Maturitas* 2016; 85: 88–95

Jacobs HS, Loeffler FE. Postmenopausal hormone replacement therapy. *BMJ* 1992; 305(6866): 1403–1408

Kotsopoulos J, Huzarski T, Gronwald J, et al. Hormone replacement therapy after menopause and risk of breast cancer in BRCA1 mutation carriers: a case-control study. *Breast Cancer Research and Treatment* 2016; 155(2): 365–373

Lee JY, Park YK, Cho KH, et al. Suicidal ideation among postmenopausal women on hormone replacement therapy: the Korean National Health and Nutrition Examination Survey (KNHANES V) from 2010 to 2012. *Journal of Affective Disorders* 2016; 189: 214–219

Li C, Wang L, Sun X, et al. Analysis of the long-term beneficial effects of menopausal hormone therapy on sleep quality and menopausal symptoms. *Experimental and Therapeutic Medicine* 2019; 18(5): 3905–3912

Liu Y, Ma L, Yang X, et al. Menopausal hormone replacement therapy and the risk of ovarian cancer: a meta-analysis. *Frontiers in Endocrinology* 2019; Dec 3 10:801

Lock M. Contested meanings of the menopause. *Lancet* 1991; 337(8752): 1270–1272

Lupo M, Dains JE, Madsen LT. Hormone replacement therapy: an increased risk of recurrence and mortality for breast cancer patients? *Journal of the Advanced Practitioner in Oncology* 2015; 6(4): 322–330

Magraith K, Stuckey B. Making choices at menopause. *Australian Journal of General Practice* 2019; 48(7): 457–462

Maki PM, Girard LM, Manson JE. Menopausal hormone therapy and cognition. *BMJ* 2019; Mar 6 364: l877

Manson JE, Chlebowski RT, Stefanick ML, et al. Menopausal hormone therapy and health outcomes during the intervention and extended poststopping phases of the Women's Health Initiative randomized trials. *JAMA* 2013; 310(13): 1353–1368

Manson JE, Kaunitz AM. Menopause management: getting clinical care back on track. *New England Journal of Medicine* 2016; 374(9): 803–806

Minkin MJ. Menopause: hormones, lifestyle, and optimizing aging. *Obstetrics and Gynecology Clinics of North America* 2019; 46(3): 501–514

Naftolin F, Friedenthal J, Nachtigall R, et al. Cardiovascular health and the menopausal woman: the role of estrogen and when to begin and end hormone treatment. F1000Research 2019; Sep 3: 8

National Association for Health and Care Excellence (NICE). Menopause: diagnosis and management. NG23 November 2015

Paschou SA, Papanas N. Type 2 diabetes mellitus and menopausal hormone therapy: an update. *Diabetes Therapy* 2019; 10(6): 2313–2320

Pinkerton JV, Conner EA, Kaunitz AM. Management of menopause and the role for hormone therapy. *Clinical Obstetrics and Gynecology* 2019; 62(4) 677–686

Pizot C, Boniol M, Mullie P, et al. Physical activity, hormone replacement therapy and breast cancer risk: a meta-analysis of prospective studies. *European Journal of Cancer* 2016; 52: 138–154

Rees M. Menopause: women should not suffer in silence. *Maturitas* 2019; 124: 91–92

Reid RL. Hormone therapy and breast cancer: risk communication and the "perfect storm." *Climacteric* 2019; 22(1): 13–16

Renoux C, Suissa S. Hormone therapy administration in postmenopausal women and risk of stroke. *Women's Health* 2011; 7(3): 355–361

Riemma G, Schiattarella A, La Verde M, et al. Efficacy of low-dose paroxetine for the treatment of hot flushes in surgical and physiological postmenopausal women: systematic review and meta-analysis of randomized trials. *Medicina* 2019; Aug 31: 55(9)

Royal College of Obstetrics and Gynaecology. *Scientific Advisory Committee Opinion Paper 6: alternatives to HRT for management of symptoms of the menopause.* London: RCOG, May 2006

Rossouw JE, Anderson GL, Prentice RL (Division of Women's Health Initiative). Risks and benefits of estrogen plus progestin in healthy postmenopausal women: principal results from the Women's Health Initiative randomized controlled trial. *JAMA* 2002; 288(3): 321–323

Santen RJ, Stuenkel CA, Burger HG, et al. Competency in menopause management: whither goest the internist? *Journal of Women's Health* 2014; 23(4): 281–285

Song Y, Xu W, Chatooah ND, et al. Comparison of low dose versus ultra-low dose hormone therapy in menopausal symptoms and quality of life in perimenopausal women. *Gynecological Endocrinology* 2020 Mar; 36(3): 252–256

Stepan JJ, Hruskova H, Kverka M. Update on menopausal hormone therapy for fracture prevention. *Current Osteoporosis Reports* 2019; 17(6): 465–473

Stuenkel CG, Davis SR, Gompel A, et al. Treatment of symptoms of the menopause: an Endocrine Society clinical practice guideline. *Journal of Clinical Endocrinology and Metabolism* 2015; 100(11): 281–285

Stute P, Spyropoulou A, Karageorgiou V, et al. Management of depressive symptoms in peri- and postmenopausal women: EMAS position statement. *Maturitas* 2020; 131: 91–101

Tackett AH, Bailey AL, Foody JM, et al. Hormone replacement therapy among postmenopausal women presenting with acute myocardial infarction: insights from the GUSTO-III trial. *American Heart Journal* 2010; 160(4): 687–684

Whayne TF, Mukherjee D. Women, the menopause, hormone replacement therapy and coronary heart disease. *Current Opinion in Cardiology* 2015; 30(4): 432–438

Zbuk K, Anand SS. Declining incidence of breast cancer after decreased use of hormone replacement therapy: magnitude and time lags in different countries. *Journal of Epidemiology and Community Health* 2012; 66(1): 1–7

Natural Menopause

Borba CM, Ferreira CF, Ferreira FV, et al. Effect of sulpiride on menopausal hot flashes: a randomized, double-blind, placebo-controlled clinical trial. *Gynecological Endocrinology* 2020 Mar; 36(3): 247–251

Caretto M, Giannini A, Simoncini T. An integrated approach to diagnosing and managing sleep disorders in menopausal women. *Maturitas* 2019; 128: 1–3

Chiechi LM, Putignano G, Guerra V, et al. The effect of a soy rich diet on the vaginal epithelium in post menopause: a randomized double blind trial. *Maturitas* 2003; 45(4): 241–246

Hachul H, Tufik S. Hot flashes: treating the mind, body, and soul. *Menopause* 2019; 26(5): 461–462

Komesaroff PA, Black CV, Cable V, et al. Effects of wild yam extract on menopausal symptoms, lipids and sex hormones in healthy postmenopausal women. *Climacteric* 2001; 4(2): 144–1450

Lee J, Han Y, Cho HH, et al. Sleep disorders and menopause. *Journal of Menopausal Medicine* 2019; 25(2): 83–876

Morelli V, Naquin C. Alternative therapies for traditional disease states: menopause. *American Family Physician* 2002; 66(1): 129–134

Nachtigall LE, Nachtigall L. Menopause and the gastrointestinal system: our gut feelings. *Menopause* 2019; 26(5): 459–460

National Collaborating Centre for Women's and Children's Health. Menopause: diagnosis and management. London: National Institute for Health and Care Excellence (NICE) 2015; NICE guideline 23

North American Menopause Society. Treatment of menopause-associated vasomotor symptoms: position statement of the North American Menopause Society. *Menopause* 2004; 11(1): 11–33

Uesugi T, Toda T, Okuhira T, et al. Evidence of estrogenic effect by the three-month-intervention of isoflavone on vaginal maturation and bone metabolism in early postmenopausal women. *Endocrine Journal* 2003; 50(5): 613–619

Wilcox G, Wahlqvist ML, Burger HG, et al. Oestrogenic effects of plant foods in postmenopausal women. *BMJ* 1990; 301(6757): 905–906

Zhu D, Chung HF, Dobson AJ, et al. Age at natural menopause and risk of incident cardiovascular disease: a pooled analysis of individual patient data. *Lancet Public Health* 2019; 4(11): e553–e564

Phytoestrogens

Adlercreutz H, Hamalainen E, Gorbach S, et al. Dietary phyto-estrogens and the menopause in Japan. *Lancet* 1992; 339(8803): 1233

Agosta C, Atlante M, Benvenuti C. Randomized controlled study on clinical efficacy of isoflavones plus *Lactobacillus sporogenes*, associated or not with a natural anxiolytic agent in menopause. *Minerva Ginecologica* 2011; 63(1): 11–17

Atteritano M, Mazzaferro S, A Bitto, et al. Genistein effects on quality of life and depression symptoms in osteopenic postmenopausal women: a two-year randomized double-blind controlled study. *Osteoporosis International* 2014; 25(3): 1123–1129

Bitto A, Granese R, Triolo O, et al. Genistein aglycone: a new therapeutic approach to reduce endometrial hyperplasia. *Phytomedicine* 2010; 17(11): 844–850

Chen LR, Ko NY, Chen KH. Isoflavone supplements for menopausal women: a systematic review. *Nutrients* 2019; 11(11): pii: E2649

Cheng PR, Chen JJ, Zhou XY, et al. Do soy isoflavones improve cognitive function in postmenopausal women? A meta-analysis. *Menopause* 2015; 22(2): 198–206

Cianci A, Colacurci N, Paoletti AM, et al. Soy isoflavones, inulin, calcium, and vitamin D3 in post-menopausal hot flushes: an observational study. *Clinical and Experimental Obstetrics and Gynecology* 2015; 42(6): 743–745

Cutler GJ, Nettleton JA, Ross JA, et al. Dietary flavonoid intake and risk of cancer in postmenopausal women: the Iowa Women's Health Study. *International Journal of Cancer* 2008; 123(3): 664–671

Daily KW, Ko BS, Ryuk J, et al. Equol decreases hot flashes in postmenopausal women: a systematic review and meta-analysis of randomized clinical trials. *Journal of Medicinal Food* 2019; 22(2): 127–139

Desmawati D, Sulastri D. Phytoestrogens and their health effect. *Macedonian Journal of Medical Sciences* 2019; 7(3): 495–499

Dizavandi FR, Ghazanfarpour M, Roozbeh N, et al. An overview of the phytoestrogen effect on vaginal health and dyspareunia in peri- and post-menopausal women. *Post Reproductive Health* 2019; 25(1): 11–20

Estrella RE, Landa AL, Lafuente JV, et al. Effects of antidepressants and soybean association in depressive menopausal women. *Acta Polonia Pharmaceutica* 2014; 71(2): 323–327

European Food Safety Authority. Risk assessment for peri- and post-menopausal women taking food supplements containing isolated isoflavones. *EFSA Journal* 2015; Oct 21 EFSA Journal 2015; 13(10): 4246

Faure ED, Chantre P, Mares P. Effects of a standardized soy extract on hot flushes: a multicenter, double-blind, randomized, placebo-controlled study. *Menopause* 2002; 9(5): 329–334

Fernandes ES, Celani MFS, Fistarol M, et al. Effectiveness of the short-term use of Cimicifuga racemosa in the endothelial function of postmenopausal women: a double-blind, randomized controlled trial. *Climacteric* 2020 Jun; 23(3): 245–251

Ferrari A. Soy extract phytoestrogens with high dose of isoflavones for menopausal symptoms. *Journal of Obstetrics and Gynaecology Research* 2009; 35(6):1083–1090

Ferreira LL, Silva TR, Maturana MA, et al. Dietary intake of isoflavones is associated with a lower prevalence of subclinical cardiovascular disease in postmenopausal women: cross-sectional study. *Journal of Human Nutrition and Dietetics* 2019 Dec; 32(6): 810–818

Friederichsen L, Nebel S, Zahner C, et al. Effect of Cimicifuga racemosa on metabolic parameters in women with menopausal symptoms: a retrospective observational study (CIMBOLIC). *Archives of Gynecology and Obstetrics* 2019; 2020 Feb; 301(2): 517–523

Fritz H, Seely D, Flower G, et al. Soy, red clover, and isoflavones and breast cancer: a systematic review. *PLoS One* 2013; 8(11): e81968

Hall WL, Vafeiadou K, Hallund J, et al. Soy-isoflavone-enriched foods and inflammatory biomarkers of cardiovascular disease risk in postmenopausal women: interactions with genotype and equol production. *American Journal of Clinical Nutrition* 2005; 82(6): 1260–1268

Hirose A, Terauchi M, Akiyoshi M, et al. Low-dose isoflavone aglycone alleviates psychological symptoms of menopause in Japanese women: a randomized, double-blind, placebo-controlled study. *Archives of Gynecology and Obstetrics* 2016; 293(3): 609–615

Hooper L, Ryder JJ, Kurzer MS, et al. Effects of soy protein and isoflavones on circulating hormone concentrations in pre- and post-menopausal women: a systematic review and meta-analysis. *Human Reproduction Update* 2009; 15(4): 423–440

Howes LG, Howes JB, Knight DC. Isoflavone therapy for menopausal flushes: a systematic review and meta-analysis. *Maturitas* 2006; 55(3): 203–211

Kanadys W, Baranska A, Jedrych M, et al. Effects of red clover (Trifolium pratense) isoflavones on the lipid profile of perimenopausal and postmenopausal women: a systematic review and meta-analysis. *Maturitas* 2020; 132: 7–16

Maliehe A, Ghahremani S, Kharghani S, et al. Effect of isoflavones and genistein on glucose metabolism in peri- and post-menopausal women: an overview of meta-analysis. *Journal of Menopausal Medicine* 2019; 25(2): 69–73

Mareti F, Abatzi C, Vavilis D, et al. Effect of oral phytoestrogens on endometrial thickness and breast density of perimenopausal and postmenopausal women: a systematic review and meta-analysis. *Maturitas* 2019; 124: 81–88

Mayo B, Vazquez L, Florez AB. Equol: a bacterial metabolite from the daidzein isoflavone and its presumed health benefits. *Nutrients* 2019; Sep 16 11(9): pii E2231

Mazur W. Phytoestrogen content in foods. *Baillières Clinical Endocrinology and Metabolism* 1998; 12(4): 729–742

Messina M. Soy and health update: review of the epidemiological and clinical literature. *Nutrients* 2016; 8(12) pii:E754

Messina M, Badget TM. Health effects of isoflavones misrepresented. *Food Chemistry* 2017; 225: 289–292

Messina M, Hughes C. Efficacy of soyfoods and soybean isoflavone supplements for alleviating menopausal symptoms is positively related to initial hot flush frequency. *Journal of Medicinal Food.* 2003; 6(1): 1–11

Messina M, Messina V. Provisional recommended soy protein and isoflavone intakes for healthy adults: rationale. *Nutrition Today* 2003; 38(3): 100–109

Messina M, Nagata C, Wu AH. Estimated Asian adult soy protein and isoflavone intakes. *Nutrition and Cancer* 2006; 55(1): 1–12

Miao LY, Chu TTH, Li P, et al. Cimicifuga heracleifolia is therapeutically similar to black cohosh in relieving menopausal symptoms: evidence from pharmacological and metabolomics studies. *Chinese Journal of Natural Medicine* 2019; 17(6): 435–445

Naseri R, Farnia V, Yazdchi K, et al. Comparison of Vitex agnus-castus extracts with placebo in reducing menopausal symptoms: a randomized double-blind study. *Korean Journal of Family Medicine* 2019; 40(6): 362–367

Palacios S, Pornel B, Bergeron C, et al. Endometrial safety assessment of a specific and standardized soy extract according to international guidelines. *Menopause* 2007; 14(6): 1006–1011

Palacios S, Pornel B, Vazquez F, et al. Long-term endometrial and breast safety of a specific standardized soy extract. *Climacteric* 2010; 13(4): 368–375

Palma F, Fontanesi F, Facchinetti F, et al. Acupuncture or phy(f)itoestrogens vs (e)strogen plus progestin on menopausal symptoms: a randomized study. *Gynecological Endocrinology* 2019; 35(11): 995–998

Pawlowksi J, Martin B, McCabe G, et al. Impact of equol-producing capacity and soy-isoflavone profiles of supplements on bone calcium retention in postmenopausal women: a randomized crossover trial. *American Journal of Clinical Nutrition* 2015; 102(3): 695–703

Petri NE, Nahas NJ, de Luca L, et al. Benefits of soy germ isoflavones in postmenopausal women with contraindication for conventional hormone replacement therapy. *Maturitas* 2004; 48(4): 372–380

Setchell KDR, Cole SJ. Method of defining equol-producer status and its frequency among vegetarians. *Journal of Nutrition* 2006; 136(8): 2188–2193

Simpson EE, Furlong ON, Parr HJ, et al. The effect of a randomized 12-week soy drink intervention on everyday mood in postmenopausal women. *Menopause* 2019 Mar 18 [Epub ahead of print]

Taku K, Melby MK, Kronenberg F, et al. Extract or synthesized soybean isoflavones reduce menopausal hot flash frequency and severity: systematic review and meta-analysis of randomized controlled trials. *Menopause* 2012; 19(7): 776–790

Tedeschi C, Benvenuti C. Comparison of vaginal gel isoflavones versus no topical treatment in vaginal dystrophy: results of a preliminary prospective study. *Gynecological Endocrinology* 2012; 28(8): 652–654

Thangavel P, Puga-Olguin A, Rodriguez-Landa JF, et al. Genistein as potential therapeutic candidate for menopausal symptoms and other related diseases. *Molecules* 2019; 24(21): pii: E3892

Van Erp-Baart MA, Brants HA, Kiely M, et al. Isoflavone intake in four different European countries: the VENUS approach. *British Journal of Nutrition* 2003; 89(Suppl 1): S25–30

Williamson-Hughes PS, Flickinger BD, Messina MJ, et al. Isoflavone supplements containing predominantly genistein reduce hot flash symptoms: a critical review of published studies. *Menopause* 2006; 13(5): 831–839

Zheng X, Lee SK, Chun CK. Soy isoflavones and osteoporotic bone loss: a review with an emphasis on modulation of bone remodeling. *Journal of Medicinal Food* 2016; 19(1): 1–14

Lignans

Franco OH, Burger H, Lebrun CE, et al. Higher dietary intake of lignans is associated with better cognitive performance in postmenopausal women. *Journal of Nutrition* 2005; 135(5): 1190–1195

Johnston IM, James R. *Flaxseed (linseed) oil and the power of omega-3.* New York: McGraw Hill. 1995.

Khalesi S, Irwin C, Schubert M. Flaxseed consumption may reduce blood pressure: a systematic review and meta-analysis of controlled trials. *Journal of Nutrition* 2015; 145(4): 758–765

Kreydin E, Kim M, Barrisford G, et al. Urinary lignans are associated with decreased incontinence in postmenopausal women. *Urology* 2015; 86(4): 16–20

Lemay A, Dodin S, Kadri N, et al. Flaxseed dietary supplement versus hormone replacement therapy in hypercholesterolemic menopausal women. *Obstetrics and Gynecology* 2002; 100(3): 495–504

Lowcock EC, Cotterchio M, Boucher BA. Consumption of flaxseed, a rich source of lignans, is associated with reduced breast cancer risk. *Cancer Causes and Control* 2013; 24(4): 813–816

Parikh N, Maddaford TG, Austria JA, et al. Dietary flaxseed as a strategy for improving human health. *Nutrients* 2019; 11(5). pii: E1171

Rodriguez-Garcia C, Sanchez-Quesada C, Toledo E, et al. Naturally lignan-rich foods: a dietary food for health promotion? *Molecules* 2019; 24(5): 917

Rodriguez-Leyva D, Weighell W, Edel A, et al. Potent antihypertensive action of dietary flaxseed in hypertensive patients. *Hypertension* 2013; 62(6): 1081–1089

Sacks F, Lichtenstein A, Van Horn L, et al. Soy protein, isoflavones and cardiovascular health: an American Heart Association Science Advisory for professionals from the Nutrition Committee. 504. *Circulation* 2006; 113(7): 1034–1044

Saxena S, Katare C. Evaluation of flaxseed formulation as a potential therapeutic agent in mitigation of dyslipidemia. *Biomedical Journal* 2014; 37(6): 386–390

Thompson LU, Robb P, Serraino M, et al. Mammalian lignan production from various foods. *Nutrition and Cancer* 1991; 16(1): 43–52

General Diet and Nutritional Deficiencies

Adlercreutz H, Fotsis T, Bannwart C, et al. Assay of lignans and phytoestrogens in urine of women and in cow's milk by GC/MS (SIM) In: Todd JFJ (ed), *Advances in Mass Spectrometry-85: Tenth International Mass Spectrometry Conference*. Chichester: John Wiley, 1985; 661–662

Askin M, Koc EM, Soyoz M, et al. Relationship between postmenopausal vitamin D level, menopausal symptoms and sexual functions. *Journal of the College of Physicians and Surgeons Pakistan* 2019; 29(9): 823–827

Bates B. National Diet and Nutrition Survey: results from years 5 and 6 (combined) of the rolling programme (2012/2013–2013/2014). London: TSO 2016

Campagnoli C, Abba C, Ambroggio S, et al. Polyunsaturated fatty acids (PUFAs) might reduce hot flushes: an indication from two controlled trials on soy isoflavones alone and with a PUFA supplement. *Maturitas* 2005; 51(2): 127–134

Chasapis CT, Loutsidou AC, Spiliopoulou CA, et al. Zinc and human health: an update. *Archives of Toxicology* 2012; 86: 521–534

Chedraui P, Pérez-López FR. Nutrition and health during mid-life: searching for solutions and meeting challenges for the aging population. *Climacteric* 2013; 16: 85–95

Committee on Medical Aspects of Food Policy. *Dietary Reference Values for Food Energy and Nutrients for the United Kingdom*. London: HMSO, 1991

Derbyshire E. Associations between red meat intakes and the micronutrient intake and status of UK females: a secondary analysis of the UK National Diet and Nutrition Survey. *Nutrients* 2017; 9: E768

Derbyshire E. Micronutrient intakes of British adults across mid-life: a secondary analysis of the UK National Diet and Nutrition Survey. *Frontiers in Nutrition* 2018 Jul 19; 5:55

Derbyshire EJ. *Nutrition in the childbearing years.* Chichester: Wiley-Blackwell, 2011

Ferreira T da S, Rocha TM, et al. Vitamin D deficiency is associated with insulin resistance independent of intracellular calcium, dietary calcium and serum levels of parathormone, calcitriol and calcium in premenopausal women. *Nutrición Hospitalaria* 2015; 31(4): 1491–1498

Hoeft B, Weber P, Eggersdorfer M. Micronutrients: a global perspective on intake, health benefits and economics. *International Journal for Vitamin and Nutrition Research* 2012; 82: 316–320

Hutchins AM, Lampe JW, Martini M, et al. Vegetables, fruits and legumes: effect on urinary isoflavonoid phytoestrogen and lignan excretion. *Journal of the American Dietetic Association* 1995; 95(7): 769–774

Ji X, Grandner MA, Liu J. The relationship between micronutrient status and sleep patterns: a systematic review. *Public Health Nutrition* 2017; 20: 687–701

King DE, Xiang J, Brown A. Intake of key chronic disease-related nutrients among baby boomers. *Southern Medical Journal* 2014; 107(6): 342–347

Lerchbaum E. Vitamin D and menopause: a narrative review. *Maturitas* 2014; 79(1): 3–7

Lopez-Gonzalez B, Molina-Lopez J, Florea DI, et al. Association between magnesium-deficient status and anthropometric and clinical-nutritional parameters in postmenopausal women. *Nutrición Hospitalaria* 2014; 29(3): 658–664

McCabe D, Lisy K, Lockwood C, et al. The impact of essential fatty acid, B vitamins, vitamin C, magnesium and zinc supplementation on stress levels in women: a systematic review. *JBI Database of Systematic Reviews and Implementation Reports* 2017; 15(2): 402–453

Miller R, Spiro A, Stanner S. Micronutrient status and intake in the UK: where might we be in 10 years' time? *Nutrition Bulletin* 2016; 41(1): 14–41

National Diet and Nutrition Survey. *Appendix A: Dietary Data Collection and Editing.* London: Public Health England, 2016

Nielsen FH. Magnesium deficiency and increased inflammation: current perspectives. *Journal of Inflammation Research* 2018; 11: 25–34

Olza J, Aranceta-Bartrina J, Gonzalez-Gross M, et al. Reported dietary intake and food sources of zinc, selenium, and vitamins A, E and C in the Spanish population: findings from the ANIBES Study. *Nutrients* 2017; 9: E697

Parazzini F, Di Martino M, Pellegrino P. Magnesium in the gynecological practice: a literature review. *Magnesium Research* 2017; 30(1): 1–7

Peter S, Eggersdorfer M, van Asselt D, et al. Selected nutrients and their implications for health and disease across the lifespan: a roadmap. *Nutrients* 2014; 6(12): 6076–6094

Public Health England. *Government dietary recommendations: government recommendations for energy and nutrients for males and females aged 1–18 years and 19+ years.* London: Public Health England, 2016.

Saeedian Kia A, Amani R, Cheraqhian B. The association between the risk of premenstrual syndrome and vitamin D, calcium, and magnesium status among university students: a case control study. *Health Promotion Perspectives* 2015; 5(3): 225–230

Schierbeck LL, Rejnmark L, Tofteng CL, et al. Vitamin D deficiency in postmenopausal, healthy women predicts increased cardiovascular events: a 16-year follow-up study. *European Journal of Endocrinology* 2012; 167(4): 553–560

Shamberger RJ. Calcium, magnesium, and other elements in the red blood cells and hair of normals and patients with premenstrual syndrome. *Biological Trace Element Research* 2003; 94(2): 123–129

Sherwood RA, Rocks BF, Stewart A, et al. Magnesium and the premenstrual syndrome. *Annals of Clinical Biochemistry* 1986; 23(Pt 6): 667–670

Soni M, Kos K, Lang IA, et al. Vitamin D and cognitive function. *Scandinavian Journal of Clinical and Laboratory Investigations Supplement* 2012; 243: 79–82

Wallace TC, McBurney M, Fulgoni VL III. Multivitamin/mineral supplement contribution to micronutrient intakes in the United States, 2007–2010. *Journal of the American College of Nutrition* 2014; 33(2): 94–102

White DJ, Cox KH, Peters R, et al. Effects of four-week supplementation with a multi-vitamin/mineral preparation on mood and blood biomarkers in young adults: a randomised, double-blind, placebo-controlled trial. *Nutrients* 2015; 7(11): 9005–9017

Supplements

Abdali K, Khajehei M, Tabatabaee HR. Effect of St John's wort on severity, frequency, and duration of hot flashes in premenopausal, perimenopausal and postmenopausal women: a randomized, double-blind, placebo-controlled study. *Menopause* 2010; 17(2): 326–331

Adluri RS, Zhan L, Bagchi M. Comparative effects of a novel plant-based calcium supplement with two common calcium salts on proliferation and mineralization in human osteoblast cells. *Molecular and Cellular Biochemistry* 2010; 340(1–2): 73–80

Albertazzi P, Pansini F, Bonaccorsi G, et al. The effect of dietary soy supplementation on hot flushes. *Obstetrics and Gynecology* 1998; 91(1): 6–11

Al-Dashti YA, Holt RR, Carson JG, et al. Effects of short-term dried plum (prune) intake on markers of bone resorption and vascular function in healthy postmenopausal women: a randomized crossover trial. *Journal of Medicinal Food* 2019; 22(10): 982–992

Anek A, Bunyaratavej N, Jittivilai T. Effects of short-term vitamin D supplementation on musculoskeletal and body balance for prevention of falling in postmenopausal women. *Journal of the Medical Association of Thailand* 2015; 98(Suppl 8): S26–31

Atkinson C, Warren RM, Sala E, et al. Red-clover-derived isoflavones and mammographic breast density: a double-blind, randomized, placebo-controlled trial. *Breast Cancer Research* 2004; 6(3): R170–179

Bai WP, Wang SY, Liu JL, et al. Efficacy and safety of Remifemin compared to tibolone for controlling of perimenopausal symptoms. *Zonghua fu chan ke za zhi* 2009 44(8): 597–600 [in Chinese]

Bommer S, Klein P, Suter A. First time proof of s sage's tolerability and efficacy in menopausal women with hot flushes. *Advances in Therapy* 2011; 28(6): 490–500

Borrelli F, Ernst E. Black cohosh (Cimicifuga racemosa) for menopausal symptoms: a systematic review of its efficacy. *Pharmacological Research* 2008; 58(1): 8–14

Bottari AI, Belcaro G, Ledda A, et al. Lady Prelox® improves sexual function in post-menopausal women. *Panminerva Medica* 2012; 54(1 Suppl 4): 3–9

Carter R. *Maca-Go White Paper.* San Francisco: Natural Health International, 2012

Cappelli V, Morgante G, Di Sabatino A, et al. Evaluation of the efficacy of a new nutraceutical product in the treatment of postmenopausal symptoms. *Minerva Ginecologica* 2015; 67(6): 515–521

Chen FPI, Chang CJ, Chao AS, et al. Efficacy of Femerelle for the treatment of climacteric syndrome in postmenopausal women: an open label trial. *Taiwanese Journal of Obstetrics and Gynecology* 2016; 55(3): 336–340

Dording CM, Fisher L, Papakostas G, et al. A double-blind, randomized, pilot dose-finding study of maca root (L. meyenii) for the management of SSRI-induced sexual dysfunction. *CNS Neuroscience and Therapeutics* 2008; 14(3): 182–191

Elam ML, Johnson SA, Hooshmand S, et al. A calcium-collagen chelate dietary supplement attenuates bone loss in postmenopausal women with osteopenia: a randomized controlled trial. *Journal of Medicinal Food* 2015; 18 (3): 324–331

Eliasvandi P, Khodaie L, Charandabi S, et al. Effect of a herbal capsule on chronic constipation among menopausal women: a randomised controlled trial. *Avicenna Journal of Phytomedicine* 2019; 9(6): 517–529

Ellis AC, Dudenbostel T, Crowe-White K. Watermelon juice: a novel functional food to increase circulating lycopene in older adult women. *Plant Foods for Human Nutrition* 2019; 74(2): 200–203

Erkkola R, Yang B. Sea buckthorn oils: towards healthy mucous membranes. *AgroFOOD Industry Hi-Tech* 2003; 14(3): 53–57

Gonzales G, Villaorduna L, Gasco M, et al. Maca (Lepidium meyenii Walp): a review of its biological properties. *Revista Peruana de Medicina Experimental y Salud Pública* 2014; 31(1): 100–110 [in Spanish]

Grube B, Walper A, Wheatley D. St. John's wort extract: efficacy for menopausal symptoms of psychological origin. *Advances in Therapy* 1999; 16(4): 177–186

Husband AJ. Phytoestrogens and menopause: published evidence supports a role for phytoestrogens in menopause. *BMJ* 2002; 324(7328): 52

Husband AJ. Red clover isoflavone supplements: safety and pharmacokinetics. *Journal of the British Menopause Society* 2001; Suppl. 1: 4–7

Jeri AR. The use of an isoflavone supplement to relieve hot flushes. *Female Patient* 2002; 27: 35–37.

Jiang K, Jin Y, Huang L, et al. Black cohosh improves objective sleep in postmenopausal women with sleep disturbance. *Climacteric* 2015; 18(4): 559–567

Kaats GR, Preuss HG, Stohs S, et al. A 7-year longitudinal trial of the safety and efficacy of a vitamin/ mineral enhanced plant-sourced calcium supplement. *Journal of the American College of Nutrition* 2016; 35(2): 91–99

Kanadys WM, Leszczy ska-Gorzelak B, Oleszczuk J. Efficacy and safety of Black cohosh (Actaea/ Cimicifuga racemosa) in the treatment of vasomotor symptoms: review of clinical trials. *Ginekologia Polska* 2008; 79(4): 287–296

Kargozar R, Azizi H, Salari R. A review of effective herbal medicines in controlling menopausal symptoms. *Electronic Physician* 2017; 9(11): 5826–5833

Kargozar R, Salari R, Jarahi L, et al. Urtica dioica in comparison with placebo and acupuncture: a new possibility for menopausal hot flashes: a randomized clinical trial. *Complementary Therapies in Medicine* 2019; 44: 166–173

Labos G, Trakakis E, Pliatsika P, et al. Efficacy and safety of DT56a compared to hormone therapy in Greek post-menopausal women. *Journal of Endocrinological Investigation* 2013; 36(7): 521–526

Lewis JR, Radavelli-Bagatini S, Rejnmark L, et al. The effects of calcium supplementation on verified coronary heart disease hospitalization and death in postmenopausal women: a collaborative meta-analysis of randomized controlled trials. *Journal of Bone and Mineral Research* 2015; 30(1): 165–175

Liu YR, Jiang YL, Huang RQ, et al. Hypericum perforatum L. preparations for menopause: a meta-analysis of efficacy and safety. *Climacteric* 2014; 17(4): 325–335

Lopez-Baena MT, Perez-Roncero GR, Perez-Lopez FR, et al. Vitamin D, menopause and aging: quo vadis? *Climacteric* 2020 Apr; 23(2):123–129

Manson JE, Bassuk SS. Calcium supplements: do they help or harm? *Menopause* 2014; 21(1): 106–108

Mehrpooya M, Rabiee S, Larki-Harchegani A, et al. A comparative study on the effect of "black cohosh" and "evening primrose oil" on menopausal hot flashes. *Journal of Education and Health Promotion* 2018; 7:36.

Meissner HO, Kapczynski W, Mscisz A. Use of gelatinized Maca (Maca-GO) (Lepidium peruvianum) in early postmenopausal women: a pilot study. *International Journal of Biomedical Science* 2005; 1(1): 33–45

Meissner HO, Mscisz A, Reich-Bilinska H. Hormone-balancing effect of pre-gelatinized organic Maca (Maca-GO) (Lepidium peruvianum Chacon): (II). Physiological and symptomatic responses of early-postmenopausal women to standardized doses of maca in double-blind, randomized placebo-controlled, multicenter clinical study. *International Journal of Biomedical Science* 2006; 2(4): 360–374

Meissner HO, Mscisz A, Reich-Bilinska H. Hormone-balancing effect of pre-gelatinized organic Maca (Maca-GO) (Lepidium peruvianum Chacon): (III). Clinical responses of early-postmenopausal women to Maca in double-blind, randomized, placebo-controlled, crossover configuration, outpatient study. *International Journal of Biomedical Science* 2006; 2(4): 375–394

Meissner HO, Reich-Bilinska H, Kedzia A. Pre-gelatinized Maca (Maca-GO) (Lepidium peruvianum Chacon) as non-hormonal herbal remedy to reduce menopausal symptoms in pre- and postmenopausal women. *Basic and Clinical Pharmacology and Toxicology* 2005; 97(Suppl 1) 48

Meissner HO, Reich-Bilinska H, Mscisz A. Therapeutic effect of Lepidium peruvanium Chacon (Maca-CO) used as a non-hormonal alternative to HRT in perimenopausal women – clinical pilot study. *International Journal of Biomedical Science* 2006; 2(2):143–159

Mohammad-Alizadeh-Charandabi S, Shahnazi M, Nahaee J, et al. Efficacy of black cohosh (Cimicifuga racemosa L.) in treating early symptoms of menopause: a randomized clinical trial. *Chinese Medicine* 2013; 8(1): 20

Myers SP, Vigar V. Effects of a standardised extract of Trifolium pratense (Promensil) at a dosage of 80mg in the treatment of menopausal hot flushes: a systematic review and meta-analysis. *Phytomedicine* 2017; 24: 141–147

Nachtigall LB, Nachtigall MJ, Nachtigall LE. Non-prescription alternatives to hormone replacement therapy. *Female Patient* 1999; 24(6): 59

Naseri R, Farnia V, Yasdchi K, et al. Comparison of Vitex agnus-castus extracts with placebo in reducing menopausal symptoms: a randomized double-blind study. *Korean Journal of Family Medicine* 2019; May 9 [Epub ahead of print]

Obi N, Chang-Claude J, Berger J, et al. The use of herbal preparation to alleviate climacteric disorders and risk of postmenopausal breast cancer in a German case-control study. *Cancer Epidemiology, Biomarkers and Prevention* 2009; 8(8): 2207–2213

Park H, Qin R, Smith TJ, et al. North Central Cancer Treatment Group N10C2 (Alliance): a double-blind placebo-controlled study of magnesium supplements to reduce menopausal hot flashes. *Menopause* 2015; 22(6): 627–632

Park SY, Kim HJ, Lee SR, et al. Black cohosh inhibits 17β-estradiol-induced cell proliferation of endometrial adenocarcinoma cells. *Gynecological Endocrinology* 2016; 32(10): 840–843

Peng CC, Liu CY, Kuo NR, et al. Effects of phytoestrogen supplement on quality of life of postmenopausal women: a systematic review and meta-analysis of randomized controlled trials. *Evidence-Based Complementary and Alternative Medicine* 2019 Apr 1: 3261280

Ross SM. Efficacy of a standardized isopropanolic black cohosh (Actaea racemosa) extract in treatment of uterine fibroids in comparison with tibolone among patients with menopausal symptoms. *Holistic Nursing Practice* 2014; 28(6): 386–391

Ruhlen RL, Haubner J, Tracy JK, et al. Black cohosh does not exert an estrogenic effect on the breast. *Nutrition and Cancer* 2007; 59(2): 269–277

Sánchez-Borrego R, Mendoza N, Llaneza P. A prospective study of DT56a (Femarelle®) for the treatment of menopause symptoms. *Climacteric* 2015; 18(6): 813–816

Shams T, Setia MS, Hemmings R, et al. Efficacy of black cohosh–containing preparations on menopausal symptoms: a meta-analysis. *Alternative Therapies in Health and Medicine* 2010; 16(1): 36–44

Sharif SN, Darsareh F. Impact of evening primrose oil consumption on psychological symptoms of postmenopausal women: a randomized double-blinded placebo-controlled trial. *Menopause* 2020 Feb; 27(2): 194–198

Sharif SN, Darsareh F. Effect of royal jelly on menopausal symptoms: A randomized placebo-controlled clinical trial. *Complementary Therapies in Clinical Practice* 2019; 37: 47–50

Suwanvesh NI, Manonai J, Sophonsritsuk A, et al. Comparison of Pueraria mirifica gel and conjugated equine estrogen cream effects on vaginal health in postmenopausal women. *Menopause* 2017; 24(2): 210–215

Taavoni S, Nazem Ekbatani N, Haghani H. Valerian/lemon balm use for sleep disorders during menopause. *Complementary Therapies in Clinical Practice* 2013; 19(4): 193–196

Teschke R, Bahre R, Fuchs J, et al. Black cohosh hepatotoxicity: quantitative causality evaluation in nine suspected cases. *Menopause* 2009; 16(5): 956–965

Thomas AG, Ismail R, Taylor-Swanson L, et al. Effects of isoflavones and amino acid therapies for hot flashes and co-occurring symptoms during the menopausal transitions and early postmenopause: a systematic review. *Maturitas* 2014; 78(4): 263–276

Van de Weijer PH, Barentsen R. Isoflavones from red clover (Promensil) significantly reduce menopausal hot flush symptoms compared with placebo. *Maturitas* 2002; 42(3): 187–119

Woods R, Whitehead M. Effects of red clover isoflavones (Promensil) versus placebo on uterine endometrium, vaginal maturation index and the uterine artery in healthy postmenopausal women. *Journal of the British Menopause Society* 2003; Suppl S2: 33

Yang B. *Lipophilic components of sea buckthorn (Hippophaë rhamnoides) seeds and berries and physiological effects of sea buckthorn oils.* Turku, Finland: University of Turku, 2001

Yang B, Kallio H. Composition and physiological effects of sea buckthorn lipids. *Trends in Food Science and Technology* 2002; 13(5): 160–167

Yang B, Kallio H. Physiological effects of sea buckthorn (Hippophaë rhamnoides) fruit pulp and seed oils. In: Singh V, Yang B, Kallio H, et al. (eds). *Seabuckthorn (Hippophaë L). A multipurpose wonder plant. Vol II: Biochemistry and Pharmacology.* New Delhi: Dya Publishing House, 2008, 363–389

Yang B, Kallio HP. Fatty acid composition of lipids in sea buckthorn (Hippophaë rhamnoides L.) berries of different origins. *Journal of Agricultural and Food Chemistry* 2001; 49(4): 1939–1947

Zhang Y, Yu L, Jin W, et al. Effect of ethanolic extract of *Lepidium meyenii* Walp on serum hormone levels in ovariectomized rats. *Indian Journal of Pharmacology* 2014; 46 (4); 416–419

Zheng Y, Zhu J, Zhou M, et al. Meta-analysis of long-term vitamin D supplementation on overall mortality. *PLoS One* 2013; 8 (12): e82109

Exercise and Relaxation

Aibar-Alamazán A, Hita-Contreras F, Cruz-Diaz D, et al. Effects of Pilates training on sleep quality, anxiety, depression and fatigue in postmenopausal women: a randomized controlled trial. *Maturitas* 2019; 124: 62–67

Angin E, Erden A, Can F. The effects of clinical Pilates exercises on bone mineral density, physical performance and quality of life in women with postmenopausal osteoporosis. *Journal of Back and Musculoskeletal Rehabilitation* 2015; 28(4): 849–858

Bergamin M, Gobbo S, Bullo V, et al. Effects of a Pilates exercise program on muscle strength, postural control and body composition: results from a pilot study in a group of post-menopausal women. *Age (Dordr)*. 2015; 37(6): 118

Berin E, Hammar M, Lindblom H, et al. Resistance training for hot flushes in postmenopausal women: a randomised controlled trial. *Maturitas* 2019; 126: 55–60

Blümel JE, Fica J, Chedraui P, et al. Sedentary lifestyle in middle-aged women is associated with severe menopausal symptoms and obesity. *Menopause* 2016; 23(5): 488–493

Boutcher YN, Boutcher SH, Yoo HY, et al. The effect of sprint interval training on body composition of postmenopausal women. *Medicine and Science in Sports and Exercise* 2019; 51(7): 1413–1419

Carmody JF, Crawford S, Salmoirago-Blotcher E, et al. Mindfulness training for coping with hot flashes: results of a randomized trial. *Menopause* 2011; 18(6): 611–620

Chattha R, Raghuram N, Venkatram P, et al. Treating the climacteric symptoms in Indian women with an integrated approach to yoga therapy: a randomized control study. *Menopause* 2008; 15(5): 862–870

Clond M. Emotional freedom techniques for anxiety: a systematic review with meta-analysis. *Journal of Nervous and Mental Disorders* 2016; 204(5): 388–395

Cowan MM, Gregory LW. Responses of pre- and postmenopausal females to aerobic conditioning. *Medicine and Science in Sports and Exercise* 1985; 17(1): 138–143

Crowe BM, van Puymbroeck M. Enhancing problem- and emotion-focused coping in menopausal women through yoga. *International Journal of Yoga Therapy* 2019; 29(1): 57–64

Cruz-Díaz D, Martínez-Amat A, Osuna-Pérez MC, et al. Short- and long-term effects of a six-week clinical Pilates program in addition to physical therapy on postmenopausal women with chronic low back pain: a randomized controlled trial. *Disability and Rehabilitation* 2016; 38(13): 1300–1308

Dabrowska-Galas M, Dabrowska J, Ptaszkowski K, et al. High physical activity level may reduce menopausal symptoms. *Medicina* 2019; 2019 Aug 11; 55(8): 466

Gliemann L, Hellsten Y. The exercise timing hypothesis: can exercise training compensate for the reduction in blood vessel function after menopause if timed right? *Journal of Physiology* 2019; 597(19): 4915–4925

Greist JH, Klein MH, Eischens RR, et al. Running as treatment for depression. *Comprehensive Psychiatry* 1979; 20(1): 41–54

Green SM, Key BL, McCabe RE. Cognitive-behavioral, behavioral, and mindfulness-based therapies for menopausal depression: a review. *Maturitas* 2015; 80(1): 37–47

Greendale GA, Gold GB. Lifestyle factors: are they related to vasomotor symptoms and do they modify the effectiveness or side effects of hormone therapy? *American Journal of Medicine* 2005; 118(Suppl 12B): 148–154

Hita-Contreras F, Martínez-Amat A, Cruz-Díaz D, et al. Fall prevention in postmenopausal women: the role of Pilates exercise training. *Climacteric* 2016; 19(3): 229–233

Ho TY, Redmayne GP, Tran A, et al. The effect of interval sprinting exercise on vascular function and aerobic fitness of post-menopausal women. *Scandinavian Journal of Medicine and Science in Sports* 2020 Feb; 30(2): 312–321

Hupin D, Roche F, Edouard P. Even a low-dose of moderate-to-vigorous physical activity reduces mortality by 22% in adults aged ≥60 years: a systematic review and meta-analysis. *British Journal of Sports Medicine* 2015; 49: 1262–1267

Ivarsson T, Spetz AL, Hammar M. Physical exercise and vasomotor symptoms in postmenopausal women. *Maturitas* 1998; 29(2): 139–146

Janhnke R, Larkey L, Rogers C, et al. A comprehensive review of health benefits of qigong and tai chi. *American Journal of Health Promotion* 2010; 24(6): e1–e25

Lindh-Astrand L, Nedstrand E, Wyon Y, et al. Vasomotor symptoms and quality of life in previously sedentary postmenopausal women randomised to physical activity or estrogen therapy. *Maturitas* 2004; 48(2): 97–105

Mansikkamäki K, Raitanen J, Malila N, et al. Physical activity and menopause-related quality of life: a population-based cross-sectional study. *Maturitas* 2015; 80(1): 69–74

Martin D, Notelovitz M. Effects of aerobic training on bone mineral density of postmenopausal women. *Journal of Bone and Mineral Research* 1993; 8(8): 931–936

Martires J, Zeidler M. The value of mindfulness meditation in the treatment of insomnia. *Current Opinion in Pulmonary Medicine* 2015; 21(6); 547–552

Miles C, Tait E, Schure M, et al. Effect of laughter yoga on psychological well-being and physiological measures. *Advances in Mind-Body Medicine* 2016; 30(1): 12–20

Mohr M, Helge EW, Petersen LF. Effects of soccer vs swim training on bone formation in sedentary middle-aged women. *European Journal of Applied Physiology* 2015; 115(12): 2671–2679

Nedstrand E, Wijma K, Wyon Y, et al. Applied relaxation and oral estradiol treatment of vasomotor symptoms in postmenopausal women. *Maturitas* 2005; 51(2): 154–162

Nunes PRP, Martins FM, Souza AP, et al. Comparative effects of high-intensity interval training with combined training on physical function markers in obese postmenopausal women: a randomized controlled trial. *Menopause* 2019; 26(11): 1242–1249

Vaze N, Joshi S. Yoga and menopausal transition. *Journal of Midlife Health.* 2010; 1(2): 56–58

Vidoni ED, Johnson DK, Morris JK, et al. Dose-response of aerobic exercise on cognition: a community-based, pilot randomized controlled trial. *PLoS One* 2015; 10(7): e0131647

Wang C. Comparative effectiveness of tai chi versus physical therapy in treating knee osteoarthritis: a randomized single-blind trial. American College of Rheumatology Annual Meeting, 2015.

Wen HJ, Huang T, Li T, et al. Effects of short-term step aerobics exercise on bone metabolism and functional fitness in postmenopausal women with low bone mass. *Osteoporosis International* 2017 Feb; 28(2): 539–547

Wilson PB. Perceived life stress and anxiety correlate with chronic gastrointestinal symptoms in runners. *Journal of Sports Science* 2018; 36(15): 1713–1719

Complementary Therapies

Abedian Z, Eskandari L, Abdi H, et al. The effect of acupressure on sleep quality in menopausal women: a randomized control trial. *Iranian Journal of Medical Sciences* 2015; 40(4): 328–334

Andrade DC, Carmona F, Angelucci MA, et al. Effect of a homeopathic medicine of Capsicum frutescens L. (Solanaceae) in the treatment of hot flashes in menopausal women: a phase 2 randomized controlled trial. *Homeopathy* 2019; 108(2): 102–107

Baccetti S, Da Frè M, Becorpi A, et al. Acupuncture and traditional Chinese medicine for hot flushes in menopause: a randomized trial. *Journal of Alternative and Complementary Medicine* 2014; 20(7): 550–557

Bakhtiari S, Paki S, Khalili A, et al. Effect of lavender aromatherapy through inhalation on quality of life among postmenopausal women covered by a governmental health center in Isfahan, Iran: a single-blind clinical trial. *Complementary Therapies in Clinical Practice* 2019; 34: 46–50

Bordet MF, Colas A, Marijnen P, et al. Treating hot flushes in menopausal women with homeopathic treatment: results of an observational study. *Homeopathy* 2008; 97(1): 10–15

Chiu HY, Hsieh YJ, Tsai PS. Acupuncture to reduce sleep disturbances in perimenopausal and postmenopausal women: a systematic review and meta-analysis. *Obstetrics and Gynecology* 2016; 127(3): 507–515

Darsareh F, Taavoni S, Joolaee S, et al. Effect of aromatherapy massage on menopausal symptoms: a randomized placebo-controlled clinical trial. *Menopause* 2012; 19(9): 995–999

Di YM, Yang L, Shergis JL, et al. Clinical evidence of Chinese medicine therapies for depression in women during perimenopause and menopause. *Complementary Therapies in Medicine* 2019; 49:102071

Drake CL, Kalmbach DA, Arnedt JT, et al. Treating chronic insomnia in postmenopausal women: a randomized clinical trial comparing cognitive-behavioral therapy for insomnia, sleep restriction therapy, and sleep hygiene education. *Sleep* 2019; Feb 1 43(2)

Eatemadnia A, Ansari S, Abedi P, et al. The effect of Hypericum perforatum on postmenopausal symptoms and depression. *Complementary Therapies in Medicine* 2019; 45: 109–113

Elkins GR, Fisher WI, Johnson AK, et al. Clinical hypnosis in the treatment of postmenopausal hot flashes: a randomized controlled trial. *Menopause* 2013; 20(3): 291–298

Feng J, Wang W, Zhong Y, et al. Acupuncture for perimenopausal depressive disorder: a systematic review and meta-analysis protocol. *Medicine* 2019; Feb 98(7): e14574

Ghorbani Z, Mirghafourvand M, Charandabi SM, et al. The effect of ginseng on sexual dysfunction in menopausal women: A double-blind, randomized controlled trial. *Complementary Therapies in Medicine* 2019; 45: 57–64

Green SM, Donegan E, Frey BN, et al. Cognitive behavior therapy for menopausal symptoms (CBT-Meno): a randomized controlled trial. *Menopause* 2019; 26(9): 972–980

Johnson A, Roberts L, Elkins G. Complementary and alternative medicine for menopause. *Journal of Evidence-Based Integrative Medicine* 2019; 24

Kalmbach DA, Cheng P, Arnedt JT, et al. Treating insomnia improves depression, maladaptive thinking and hyperarousal in postmenopausal women: comparing cognitive-behavioral therapy for insomnia (CBTI), sleep restriction therapy, and sleep hygiene education. *Sleep Medicine* 2019; 55: 124–134

Lund KS, Siersma V, Brodersen J, et al. Efficacy of a standardised acupuncture approach for women with bothersome menopausal symptoms: a pragmatic randomised study in primary care (the ACOM study). *BMJ Open* 2019; Feb 19 9(1): e023637

Mahdavipour F, Rahemi Z, Sadat Z, et al. The effects of foot reflexology on depression during menopause: a randomized controlled clinical trial. *Complementary Therapies in Medicine* 2019; Dec 47: 102195.

McGuire A, Anderson D. Yoga and acupuncture versus "sham" treatments for menopausal hot flashes: how do they compare? *Menopause* 2019; Apr 26(4): 337

Molefi-Youri W. Is there a role for mindfulness-based interventions (here defined as MBCT and MBSR)? *Post Reproductive Health* 2019 Sep; 25(3): 143–149

Mollaahmadi L, Keramat A, Changizi N, et al. Evaluation and comparison of the effects of various cognitive-behavioral therapy methods on climacteric symptoms: a systematic review study. *Journal of the Turkish German Gynecological Association* 2019 Aug 28; 20(3): 178–195

Nedeljkovic M, Tian L, Ji P, et al. Effects of acupuncture and Chinese herbal medicine (zhi mu 14) on hot flushes and quality of life in postmenopausal women: results of a four-arm randomized controlled pilot trial. *Menopause* 2014; 21(1): 15–24

North American Menopause Society. Clinical care recommendations: complementary and alternative medicine. https://www.menopause.org/publications/clinical-care-recommendations /chapter-6-complementary-and-alternative-medicine

North American Menopause Society. Cognitive behavior therapy shown to improve multiple menopause symptoms. May 29 2019. https://www.menopause.org/docs/default-source/press-release/cognitive -behavior-therapy-for-menopause-symptoms-5-29-19.pdf

Palma F, Fontanesi F, Facchinetti F, et al. Acupuncture or phyto(f)utiestrogens vs (e)estrogen plus progestin on menopausal symptoms: a randomized study. *Gynecological Endocrinology* 2019 Nov; 35(11): 995–998

Rees M. Complementary and integrative therapies for menopause. *Complementary Therapies in Medicine* 2019; 42: 149–150

Roozbeh N, Ghazanfarpour M, Khadivzadeh T, et al. Effect of lavender on sleep, sexual desire, vasomotor, psychological and physical symptoms among menopausal and elderly women: a systematic review. *Journal of Menopausal Medicine* 2019; 25(2): 88–93

Van der Sluijs CP, Bensoussan A, Livanage L, et al. Women's health during mid-life survey: the use of complementary and alternative medicine by symptomatic women transitioning through menopause in Sydney. *Menopause* 2007; 14(3): 397–403

Van Driel CM, Stuursma A, Schoevers MJ, et al. Mindfulness, cognitive behavioural and behaviour-based therapy for natural and treatment-induced menopausal symptoms: a systematic review and meta-analysis. *British Journal of Obstetrics and Gynaecology* 2019; 126(3): 330–339

Taavoni S, Darsareh F, Joolaee S, et al. The effect of aromatherapy massage on the psychological symptoms of postmenopausal Iranian women. *Complementary Therapies in Medicine* 2013; 21(3): 158–163

Taylor-Swanson L, Thomas A. Effects of traditional Chinese medicine on symptom clusters during the menopausal transition. *Climacteric* 2015; 18(2): 142–156

Thompson EA, Reilly D. The homeopathic approach to the treatment of symptoms of oestrogen withdrawal in breast cancer patients: a prospective observational study. *Homeopathy* 2003; 92(3): 131–134

Want Y, Lou XT, Shi YH, et al. Erxian decoction, a Chinese herbal formula, for menopausal syndrome: an updated systematic review. *Journal of Ethnopharmacology* 2019; Apr 24, 234: 8–20

Wyon Y, Wijma K, Nedstrand E, et al. A comparison of acupuncture and oral estradiol treatment of vasomotor symptoms in postmenopausal women. *Climacteric* 2004; 7(2): 153–164

Xiao X, Zhang J, Jin Y, et al. Acupuncture for perimenopausal depression: a protocol for a systematic review and meta-analysis. *Medicine* 2019; Jan 98(2): e14073

Heart Health

Abumweis SS, Jones PJ. Cholesterol-lowering effect of plant sterols. *Current Atherosclerosis Reports* 2008; 10(6): 467–472

Chen CY, Bakhiet RM, Hart V, et al. Isoflavones improve plasma homocysteine status and antioxidant defense system in healthy young men at rest but do not ameliorate oxidative stress induced by 80% VO2pk exercise. *Annals of Nutrition and Metabolism* 2005; 49(1): 33–41

Erdman JW Jr. AHA Science Advisory: Soy protein and cardiovascular disease: a statement for healthcare professionals from the Nutrition Committee of the AHA. *Circulation* 2000; 102(20): 2555–2559

Erkkila AT, Lehto S, Pyorala K, et al. n-3 fatty acids and 5-y risks of death and cardiovascular disease events in patients with coronary artery disease. *American Journal of Clinical Nutrition* 2003; 78(1): 65–71

Geleijnse JM, Giltay EJ, Grobbee DE, et al. Blood pressure response to fish oil supplementation: metaregression analysis of randomized trials. *Journal of Hypertension* 2002; 20(8): 1493–1499

Haq IU, Jackson PR, Yeo WW, et al. Sheffield risk and treatment table for cholesterol lowering for primary prevention of coronary heart disease. *Lancet* 1995; 346(8988): 1467–1471

Howes JB, Tran D, Brillante D, et al. Effects of dietary supplementation with isoflavones from red clover on ambulatory blood pressure and endothelial function in postmenopausal type 2 diabetes. *Diabetes, Obesity and Metabolism* 2003; 5(5): 325–332

Jenkins DJ, Kendall CW, Jackson CJ, et al. Effects of high- and low-isoflavone soy foods on blood lipids, oxidized LDL, homocysteine, and blood pressure in hyperlipidemic men and women. *American Journal of Clinical Nutrition* 2002; 76(2): 365–372

Jeri A. Effects of isoflavone phytoestrogens on lipid profile in postmenopausal Peruvian women. Presented at the 10th World Congress on the Menopause, Berlin, June 2002

Li SH, Liu XX, Bai YY, et al. Effect of oral isoflavone supplementation on vascular endothelial function in postmenopausal women: a meta-analysis of randomized placebo-controlled trials. *American Journal of Clinical Nutrition* 2009; 91(2): 480–486

Marchioli R, Schweiger C, Tavazzi L, et al. Efficacy of n-3 polyunsaturated fatty acids after myocardial infarction: results of GISSI-Prevenzione trial. *Lipids* 2001; 36(Suppl): S119–126

Mitsuyoshi K, Hiramatsu Y, Takata T, et al. Effects of eicosapentaenoic acid on lipid metabolism in obesity treatment. *Obesity Surgery* 1991; 1(2): 165–169

Nestel P. Fish oil fatty acids beneficially modulate vascular function. *World Review of Nutrition and Dietetics* 2001; 88: 86–89

Nestel P, Pomeroy S, Kay S, et al. Isoflavones from red clover improve systemic arterial compliance but not plasma lipids in menopausal women. *Journal of Clinical Endocrinology and Metabolism* 1999; 84(3): 895–898

Nestel P, Shige H, Pomeroy S, et al. The n-3 fatty acids eicosapentaenoic acid and docosahexaenoic acid increase systemic arterial compliance in humans. *American Journal of Clinical Nutrition* 2002; 76(2): 326–330

Okuda N, Ueshima H, Okayama A, et al. Relation of long chain n-3 polyunsaturated fatty acid intake to serum high density lipoprotein cholesterol among Japanese men in Japan and Japanese-American men in Hawaii: the interlipid study. *Atherosclerosis* 2005; 178(2): 371–379

Okumura T, Fujioka Y, Morimoto S, et al. Eicosapentaenoic acid improves endothelial function in hypertriglyceridemic subjects despite increased lipid oxidizability. *American Journal of the Medical Sciences* 2002; 324(5): 247–253

Ortega RM, Palencia A, Lopez-Sobaler AM. Improvement of cholesterol levels and reduction of cardiovascular risk via the consumption of phytosterols. *British Journal of Nutrition* 2006; 96: Suppl 1: S89–93

Rodriguez-Leyva D, Weighell W, Edel A, et al. Potent antihypertensive action of dietary flaxseed in hypertensive patients. *Hypertension* 2013; 62(6): 1081–1089

Sacks FM, Lichtenstein A, Van Horn L, et al. Soy protein, isoflavones, and cardiovascular health: an American Heart Association science advisory for professionals from the Nutrition Committee. *Circulation* 2006; 113: 1034–1044

Steinberg FM, Guthrie NL, Villablanca AC, et al. Soy protein with isoflavones has favorable effects on endothelial function that are independent of lipid and antioxidant effects in healthy postmenopausal women. *American Journal of Clinical Nutrition* 2003; 78(1): 123–130

Tagawa T, Hirooka Y, Shimokawa H, et al. Long-term treatment with eicosapentaenoic acid improves exercise-induced vasodilation in patients with coronary artery disease. *Hypertension Research* 2002; 25(6): 823–829

Taku K, Umegaki K, Sato Y, et al. Soy isoflavones lower serum total and LDL cholesterol in humans: a meta-analysis of 11 randomized controlled trials. *American Journal of Clinical Nutrition* 2007; 85(4): 1148–1156

Teede HJ, McGrath BP, de Silva L, et al. Isoflavones reduce arterial stiffness: a placebo-controlled study in men and postmenopausal women. *Arteriosclerosis, Thrombosis and Vascular Biology* 2003; 23(6): 1066–1071

Thies F, Garry JM, Yaqoob P, et al. Association of n-3 polyunsaturated fatty acids with stability of atherosclerotic plaques: a randomised controlled trial. *Lancet* 2003; 361(9356): 477–485

Von Schacky C. The role of omega-3 fatty acids in cardiovascular disease. *Current Atherosclerosis Reports* 2003; 5(2): 139–145

Washburn S, Burke GL, Morgan T, et al. Effect of soy protein supplementation on serum lipoproteins, blood pressure and menopausal symptoms in perimenopausal women. *Menopause* 1999; 6(1): 7–13

Yu Z, Zhang G, Zhao H. Effects of puerariae isoflavone on blood viscosity, thrombosis and platelet function. *Zhong yao cai* 1997; 20(9): 468–469

Zhan S, Ho SC. Meta-analysis of the effects of soy protein containing isoflavones on the lipid profile. *American Journal of Clinical Nutrition* 2005; 81(2): 397–408

Zhang YB, Chen WH, Guo JJ, et al. Soy isoflavone supplementation could reduce body weight and improve glucose metabolism in non-Asian postmenopausal women: a meta-analysis. *Nutrition* 2013; 29 (1): 8–14

Osteoporosis and Postmenopausal Health

Alekel DL, Van Loan MD, Koehler KJ, et al. The soy isoflavones for reducing bone loss (SIRBL) study: a 3-y randomized controlled trial in postmenopausal women. *American Journal of Clinical Nutrition* 2009; 91(1): 218–230

Arjmandi BH, Khalil DA, Smith BJ, et al. Soy protein has a greater effect on bone in postmenopausal women not on hormone replacement therapy, as evidenced by reducing bone resorption and urinary calcium excretion. *Journal of Clinical Endocrinology and Metabolism* 2003; 88(3): 1048–1054

Atkinson C, Compston JE, Day NE, et al. The effects of phytoestrogen isoflavones on bone density in women: a double-blind, randomized, placebo-controlled trial. *American Journal of Clinical Nutrition* 2004; 79(2): 326–333

Blumsohn A, Herrington K, Hannon RA, et al. The effect of calcium supplementation on the circadian rhythm of bone resorption. *Journal of Clinical Endocrinology and Metabolism* 1994; 79(3): 730–735

Brink E, Coxam V, Robins S, et al. Long-term consumption of isoflavone-enriched foods does not affect bone mineral density, bone metabolism, or hormonal status in early postmenopausal women: a randomized, double-blind, placebo controlled study. *American Journal of Clinical Nutrition* 2008; 87(3): 761–770

Chen YM, Ho SC, Lam SS, et al. Beneficial effect of soy isoflavones on bone mineral content was modified by years since menopause, body weight, and calcium intake: a double-blind, randomized, controlled trial. *Menopause* 2004; 11(3): 246–254.

De Bakker CMJ, Burt LA, Gabel L, et al. Associations between breastfeeding history and early postmenopausal bone loss. *Calcified Tissue International* 2020 Mar; 106(3): 264–273

Dixon AS. Non-hormonal treatment of osteoporosis. *BMJ* 1983; 286(6370): 999–1000

Ettinger B, Grady D. The waning effect of postmenopausal estrogen therapy on osteoporosis. *New England Journal of Medicine* 1993; 329(16): 1141–1146

Higgs J, Derbyshire E, Styles K. Nutrition and osteoporosis prevention for the orthopaedic surgeon: a wholefoods approach. *EFORT Open Reviews.* 2017; 2(6): 300–308

Horiuchi T, Onouchi T, Takahashi M, et al. Effect of soy protein on bone metabolism in postmenopausal Japanese women. *Osteoporosis International* 2000; 11(8): 721–724

Iwamoto J. Role of exercise and sports in the prevention of osteoporosis. *Clinical Calcium* 2017; 27 (1): 17–23

Kaats GR, Preuss HG, Stohs S, et al. A 7-year longitudinal trial of the safety and efficacy of a vitamin/mineral enhanced plant-sourced calcium supplement. *Journal of the American College of Nutrition* 2016; 35(2): 91–99

Kanis JA, Johnell O, Gullberg B, et al. Evidence for efficacy of drugs affecting bone metabolism in preventing hip fracture. *BMJ* 1992; 305(6862): 1124–1128

Kenny AM, Mangano KM, Abourizk RH, et al. Soy proteins and isoflavones affect bone mineral density in older women: a randomized controlled trial. *American Journal of Clinical Nutrition* 2009; 90: 234–242

Koh WP, Wu AH, Wang R, et al. Gender-specific associations between soy and risk of hip fracture in the Singapore Chinese Health Study. *American Journal of Epidemiology* 2009;170(7): 901–909

Ma DF, Qin LQ, Wang PY, et al. Soy isoflavone intake increases bone mineral density in the spine of menopausal women: meta-analysis of randomized controlled trials. *Clinical Nutrition* 2008; 27(1): 57–64

Marini H, Bitto A, Altavilla D, et al. Breast safety and efficacy of genistein aglycone for postmenopausal bone loss: a follow-up study. *Journal of Clinical Endocrinology and Metabolism* 2008; 93(12): 4787–4796

Marini H, Minutoli L, Polito F, et al. Effects of the phytoestrogen genistein on bone metabolism in osteopenic postmenopausal women: a randomized trial. *Annals of Internal Medicine* 2007; 146(12): 839–847

Martin D, Notelovitz M. Effects of aerobic training on bone mineral density of postmenopausal women. *Journal of Bone and Mineral Research* 1993; 8(8): 931–936

Mei J, Yeung SS, Kung AW. High dietary phytoestrogen intake is associated with higher bone mineral density in postmenopausal but not premenopausal women. *Journal of Clinical Endocrinology and Metabolism* 2001; 86(11): 5217–5221

Messina M, Messina V. Soyfoods, soybean isoflavones and bone health: a brief overview. *Journal of Renal Nutrition* 2000; 10(2): 63–68

Messina M, Ho S, Alekel DL. Skeletal benefits of soy isoflavones: a review of the clinical trial and epidemiologic data. *Current Opinion in Clinical Nutrition* 2004; 7(6): 649–658

Morabito N, Crisafulli A, Vergara C, et al. Effects of genistein and hormone-replacement therapy on bone loss in early postmenopausal women: a randomized double-blind placebo-controlled study. *Journal of Bone and Mineral Research* 2002; 17(10): 1904–1912

Morley J, Moayyeri A, Ali L, et al. Persistence and compliance with osteoporosis therapies among postmenopausal women in the UK: clinical practice research datalink. *Osteoporosis International* 2020 Mar; 31(3): 533–545

Peel N, Eastell R. Osteoporosis. *BMJ* 1995; 310(6985); 989–992

Poulsen RC, Kruger MC. Soy phytoestrogens: impact on postmenopausal bone loss and mechanisms of action. *Nutrition Reviews* 2008; 66(7): 359–374

Scheiber MD, Liu JH, Subbiah MT, et al. Dietary inclusion of whole soy foods results in significant reductions in clinical risk factors for osteoporosis and cardiovascular disease in normal postmenopausal women. *Menopause* 2001; 8(5): 384–392

Setchell KD, Lydeking-Olsen E. Dietary phytoestrogens and their effect on bone: evidence from in vitro and in vivo, human observational, and dietary intervention studies. *American Journal of Clinical Nutrition* 2003; 78(3 Suppl): 593S–609S

Studd JWW, Whitehead MI (eds). *The Menopause*. Oxford: Blackwell Scientific Publications, 1988

Tsunenari T, Yamada S, Kawakatsu M, et al. Menopause-related changes in bone mineral density in Japanese women: a longitudinal study on lumbar spine and proximal femur. *Calcified Tissue International* 1995; 56(1): 5–10

Van Papendorp DH, Coetzer H, Kruger MC. Biochemical profile of osteoporotic patients on essential fatty acid supplementation. *Nutrition Research* 1995; 15: 325–334

Vupadhyayula PM, Gallagher JC, Templin T, et al. Effects of soy protein isolate on bone mineral density and physical performance indices in postmenopausal women: a 2-year randomized, double-blind, placebo-controlled trial. *Menopause* 2009; 16(2): 320–328

Wen HJ, Huang TH, Li TL, et al. Effects of short-term step aerobics exercise on bone metabolism and functional fitness in postmenopausal women with low bone mass. *Osteoporosis International* 2017 Feb; 28(2): 539–547

WHO Study Group. *Assessment of fracture risk and its application to screening for postmenopausal osteoporosis*. Geneva: World Health Organization, 1994

Wilcox G, Wahlqvist ML, Burger HG, et al. Oestrogenic effects of plant foods in postmenopausal women. *BMJ* 1990; 301(6757): 905–906

Zhang X, Shu XO, Li H, et al. Prospective cohort study of soy food consumption and risk of bone fracture among postmenopausal women. *Archives of Internal Medicine* 2005;165(16): 1890–1895

Zheng X, Lee SK, Chun CK. Soy isoflavones and osteoporotic bone loss: a review with an emphasis on modulation of bone remodeling. *Journal of Medicinal Food* 2016; 19(1): 1–14

Memory and Cognitive Function

Atema V, Van Leeuwen M, Oldenburg HS, et al. Design of a randomized controlled trial of Internet-based cognitive behavioural therapy for treatment-induced menopausal symptoms in breast cancer survivors. *BMC Cancer*. 2016; 16(1): 920

Cheng PF, Chen JJ, Zhou XY, et al. Do soy isoflavones improve cognitive function in postmenopausal women? A meta-analysis. *Menopause* 2015; 22(2):198–206

Duffy R, Wiseman H, File SE. Improved cognitive function in postmenopausal women after 12 weeks of consumption of a soy extract containing isoflavones. *Pharmacology, Biochemistry, and Behavior* 2003; 75(3): 721–729

Elsabagh S, Hartley DE, File SE. Limited cognitive benefits in Stage +2 postmenopausal women after six weeks of treatment with Ginkgo biloba. *Journal of Psychopharmacology* 2005; 19(2): 173–179

File SE, Jarrett N, Fluck E, et al. Eating soy improves human memory. *Psychopharmacology* 2001; 157(4): 430–436

Henderson VW, St John JA, Hodia HN, et al. Long-term soy isoflavone supplementation and cognition in women: a randomized controlled trial. *Neurology* 2012; 78 (23): 1841–1848

Kritz-Silverstein D, Von Muhlen D, et al. Isoflavones and cognitive function in older women: the soy and postmenopausal health in aging (SOPHIA) study. *Menopause* 2003; 10(3): 196–202

McBride RL, Horsfield S, Sandler CX, et al. Cognitive remediation training improves performance in patients with chronic fatigue syndrome. *Psychiatry Research* 2017; 257: 400–405

Roozbeh N, Kashef R, Ghazanfarpour M, et al. Overview of the effect of herbal medicines and isoflavones on the treatment of cognitive function. *Journal of Menopausal Medicine* 2018; 24(2): 113–118

Sood R, Kuhle CL, Kapoor E, et al. Association of mindfulness and stress with menopausal symptoms in midlife women. *Climacteric* 2019; 22(4): 377–382.

Breast Health

Ballard-Barbash R, Neuhouser ML. Challenges in design and interpretation of observational research on health behaviors and cancer survival. *JAMA* 2009; 302(22): 2483–2484.

Boyd NF, Lockwood GA, Martin LJ, et al. Mammographic density as a marker of susceptibility to breast cancer: a hypothesis. *IARC Scientific Publications* 2001; 154: 163–169

Fleming RM. What effect, if any, does soy protein have on breast tissue? *Integrative Cancer Therapies* 2003; 2(3): 225–228

Goodman MT, Wilkens LR, Hankin JH, et al. Association of soy and fiber consumption with the risk of endometrial cancer. *American Journal of Epidemiology* 1997; 146(4): 294–306

Guha N, Kwan ML, Quesenberry CP, et al. Soy isoflavones and risk of cancer recurrence in a cohort of breast cancer survivors: the Life After Cancer Epidemiology study. *Breast Cancer Research and Treatment* 2009; 118(12): 395–405

Helferich WG, Andrade JE, Hoagland MS. Phytoestrogens and breast cancer: a complex story. *Inflammopharmacology* 2008; 16(5): 219–226

Horn-Ross PL, John EM, Canchola AJ, et al. Phytoestrogen intake and endometrial cancer risk. *Journal of the National Cancer Institute* 2003; 95(15): 1158–1164

Ingram DM, Hickling C, West L, et al. A double-blind randomized controlled trial of isoflavones in the treatment of cyclical mastalgia. *Breast* 2002; 11(2): 170–174

Kim HA, Jeong KS, Kim YK. Soy extract is more potent than genistein on tumor growth inhibition. *Anticancer Research* 2008; 28(5A): 2837–2841

Lee SA, Shu XO, Li H, et al. Adolescent and adult soy food intake and breast cancer risk: results from the Shanghai Women's Health Study. *American Journal of Clinical Nutrition* 2009; 89(6): 1920–1926

Lu LJ, Anderson KE, Grady JJ, et al. Decreased ovarian hormones during a soy diet: implications for breast cancer prevention. *Cancer Research* 2000; 60(15): 4112–2411

Maskarinec G, Murphy S, Franke AA, et al. The effects of a nutritional intervention with soyfoods on markers of breast cancer risk. *Experimental Biology 2004*; Abstract 728: 4

Maskarinec G, Williams AE, Carlin L. Mammographic densities in a one-year isoflavone intervention. *European Journal of Cancer Prevention* 2003; 12(2):165–169

Messina M, Hilakivi-Clarke L. Early intake appears to be the key to the proposed protective effects of soy intake against breast cancer. *Nutrition and Cancer* 2009; 61(6): 792–798

Messina M, McCaskill-Stevens W, Lampe JW. Addressing the soy and breast cancer relationship: review, commentary, and workshop proceedings. *Journal of the National Cancer Institute* 2006; 98(18): 1275–1284

Messina M, Watanabe S, Setchell KDR. Report on the 8th International Symposium on the Role of Soy in Health Promotion and Chronic Disease Prevention and Treatment. *Journal of Nutrition* Suppl: 2009 Apr; 139(4): 796S–802S

Messina M, Wood CE. Soy isoflavones, estrogen therapy, and breast cancer risk: analysis and commentary, *Nutrition Journal* 2008; 7: 17

Messina M, Wu AH. Perspectives on the soy–breast cancer relation. *American Journal of Clinical Nutrition* 2009; 89(5): 1673S–1679S

Peng JH, Zhang F, Zhang HX, et al. Prepubertal octylphenol exposure up-regulate BRCA1 expression, down-regulate ERalpha expression and reduce rat mammary tumorigenesis. *Cancer Epidemiology* 2009; 33(1): 51–55

Shu XO, Zheng Y, Cai H, et al. Soy food intake and breast cancer survival. *JAMA* 2009; 302(22): 2437–2443

Warri A, Saarinen NM, Makela S, et al. The role of early life genistein exposures in modifying breast cancer risk. *British Journal of Cancer* 2008; 98(9) 1485–1493

Wu AH, Stanczyk FZ, Seow A, et al. Soy intake and other lifestyle determinants of serum estrogen levels among postmenopausal Chinese women in Singapore. *Cancer Epidemiology Biomarkers and Prevention* 2002; 11(9): 844–851

Xu X, Duncan AM, Wangen KE, et al. Soy consumption alters endogenous estrogen metabolism in postmenopausal women. *Cancer Epidemiology Biomarkers and Prevention* 2000; 9(8): 781–786

Cancer Prevention

Beiler JS, Zhu K, Hunter S, et al. A case-control study of menstrual factors in relation to breast cancer risk in African-American women. *Journal of the National Medical Association* 2003; 95(10): 930–938

Den Tonkelaar I, de Waard F. Regularity and length of menstrual cycles in women aged 41–46 in relation to breast cancer risk: results from the DOM-project. *Breast Cancer Research and Treatment* 1996; 38(3): 253–258

Huang Y, Cao S, Nagamani M, et al. Decreased circulating levels of tumor necrosis factor alpha in postmenopausal women during consumption of soy-containing isoflavones. *Journal of Clinical Endocrinology and Metabolism* 2005; 90(7): 3956–3962

Jakes RW, Duffy SW, Ng FC, et al. Mammographic parenchymal patterns and self-reported soy intake in Singapore Chinese women. *Cancer Epidemiology Biomarkers and Prevention* 2002; 11(7): 608–613

Kumar NB, Cantor A, Allen K, et al. The specific role of isoflavones on estrogen metabolism in premenopausal women. *Cancer* 2002; 94(4): 1166–1174

Magee PJ, McGlynn H, Rowland IR. Differential effects of isoflavones and lignans on invasiveness of MDA-MB-231 breast cancer cells in vitro. *Cancer Letters* 2004; 208(1): 35–41

Peterson TG, Ji GP, Kirk M, et al. Metabolism of the isoflavones genistein and biochanin A in human breast cancer cell lines. *American Journal of Clinical Nutrition* 1998; 68(6 Suppl): 1505S–1511S

Pfeiffer E, Treiling CR, Hoehle SI, et al. Isoflavones modulate the glucuronidation of estradiol in human liver microsomes. *Carcinogenesis* 2005; 26(12): 2172–2178

Valachovicova T, Slivova V, Bergman H, et al. Soy isoflavones suppress invasiveness of breast cancer cells by the inhibition of NF-kappaB/AP-1-dependent and -independent pathways. *International Journal of Oncology* 2004; 25(5): 1389–1395

Yamamoto S, Sobue T, Kobayashi M, et al. Soy, isoflavones, and breast cancer risk in Japan. *Journal of the National Cancer Institute* 2003; 95(12): 906–913

Yin F, Giuliano AE, Van Herle AJ. Growth inhibitory effects of flavonoids in human thyroid cancer cell lines. *Thyroid* 1999; 9(4): 369–376

Thyroid Function

Bruce B, Messina M, Spiller GA. Isoflavone supplements do not affect thyroid function in iodine-replete postmenopausal women. *Journal of Medicinal Food* 2003; 6(4): 309–316

Doerge DR, Sheehan DM. Goitrogenic and estrogenic activity of soy isoflavones. *Environmental Health Perspectives* 2002; 110(Suppl 3): 349–353

Duncan AM, Merz PE, Xu X, et al. Soy isoflavones exert modest hormonal effects in premenopausal women. *Journal of Clinical Endocrinology and Metabolism* 1999; 84(1): 192–197

Duncan AM, Underhill KE, Xu X, et al. Modest hormonal effects of soy isoflavones in postmenopausal women. *Journal of Clinical Endocrinology and Metabolism* 1999; 84(10): 3479–3484

Menstrual Problems

Bryant M, Dye L, Hill C, et al. Role of phytoestrogens for menstrual cycle symptoms. *Journal of Nutrition* 2003; 134: 1282 (abstract)

Ferrante F, Fusco E, Calabresi P, et al. Phyto-oestrogens in the prophylaxis of menstrual migraine. *Clinical Neuropharmacology* 2004; 27(3): 137–140

Skin and Hair Health

Draelos ZD, Blair R, Tabor A. Oral soy supplementation and dermatology. *Cosmetic Dermatology* 2007; 20(4); 202–204

Izumi T, Makoto S, Obata A, et al. Oral intake of soy isoflavone aglycone improves the aged skin of adult women. *Journal of Nutrition Science and Vitaminology* 2007; 53(1): 57–62

Jenkins G, Wainwright LJ, Holland R, et al. Wrinkle reduction in post-menopausal women consuming a novel oral supplement: a double-blind placebo-controlled randomized study. *International Journal of Cosmetic Science* 2013; 36(1): 22–31

Le Floch C, Cheniti A, Connetable S, et al. Effect of a nutritional supplement on hair loss in women. *Journal of Cosmetic Dermatology* 2015; 14(1): 76–82

Oyama A, Ueno T, Uchiyama S, et al. The effects of natural S-equol supplementation on skin aging in postmenopausal women: a pilot randomized placebo-controlled trial. *Menopause* 2012; 19(2): 202–210

Thompson JM, Mirza MA, Park MK, et al. The role of micronutrients in alopecia areata: a review. *American Journal of Clinical Dermatology* 2017; 18(5): 663–679

Urinary Incontinence and Pelvic Floor Disorders

Badalian SS, Rosebaum PF. Vitamin D and pelvic floor disorders in women: results from the National Health and Nutrition Examination Survey. *Obstetrics and Gynecology* 2010 115(4): 795–803

Caruso S, Cianci A, Sarpietro G, et al. Ultralow 0.03mg vaginal estriol in postmenopausal women who underwent surgical treatment for stress urinary incontinence: effects on quality of life and sexual function. *Menopause* 2020 Feb; 27(2): 162–169

Dumoulin CM, Pazzoto Cacciari L, Mercier J. Keeping the pelvic floor healthy. *Climacteric* 2019; 22(3): 257–262

Elia D, Gambacciani M, Berreni N, et al. Genitourinary syndrome of menopause (GSM) and laser VEL: a review. *Hormone Molecular Biology and Clinical Investigation* 2019 Dec 19; 41(1)

Erel CT, Inan D, Mut A. Predictive factors for the efficacy of Er:YAG laser treatment of urinary incontinence. *Maturitas* 2020; 132:1–6

Franić D, Fistonic I. Laser therapy in the treatment of female urinary incontinence and genitourinary syndrome of menopause: an update. *BioMed Research International* 2019; June 4

Maniglio P, Ricciardi E, Meli F, et al. A pilot study of soft gel technology: a new vaginal device to improve the symptomatology of vulvovaginal atrophy in post-partum, menopause and in patients with recurrent vulvovaginitis. *European Review for Medical and Pharmacological Sciences* 2019; 23(14): 6035–6044

Panay N, Palacios S, Bruyniks N, et al. Symptom severity and quality of life in the management of vulvovaginal atrophy in postmenopausal women. 2019; 124: 55–61

Paraiso MFR, Ferrando CA, Sokol EF, et al. A randomized clinical trial comparing vaginal laser therapy to vaginal estrogen therapy in women with genitourinary syndrome of menopause: the VeLVET Trial. *Menopause* 2020 Jan; 27(1): 50–56

Sex

Areas F, Valadares AL, Conde DM, et al. The effect of vaginal erbium laser treatment on sexual function and vaginal health in women with a history of breast cancer and symptoms of the genitourinary syndrome of menopause: a prospective study. *Menopause* 2019 Sep; 26(9): 1052–1058

Dabrowski-Galas M, Dabrowska J, Michalski B. Sexual dysfunction in menopausal women. *Sexual Medicine* 2019; 7(4): 472–479

Eder SE. Early effect of fractional CO_2 laser treatment in post-menopausal women with vaginal atrophy. *Laser Therapy* 2018; 27(1): 41–47

Edwards D, Panay N. Treating vulvovaginal atrophy/genitourinary syndrome of menopause: how important is vaginal lubricant and moisturizer composition? *Climacteric* 2016; 1(2): 151–161

Gambacciani M, Levancini M, Cervigni M. Vaginal erbium laser: the second-generation thermotherapy for the genitourinary syndrome of menopause. *Climacteric* 2015; 18(5): 757–763

Groutz A, Ascher-Landsberg J, Lessing J, et al. Double-blind, placebo-controlled study of magnesium hydroxide for treatment of sensory urgency and detrusor instability: preliminary results. *British Journal of Obstetrics and Gynaecology* 1998; 105(6): 667–669

Mercier J, Morin M, Zaki D, et al. Pelvic floor muscle training as a treatment for genitourinary syndrome of menopause: a single-arm feasibility study. *Maturitas* 2019; Jul 125: 27–52

Nappi RE, Martini E, Cucinella L, et al. Addressing vulvovaginal atrophy (VVA)/genitourinary syndrome of menopause (GSM) for healthy aging in women. *Frontiers in Endocrinology* 2019 August 21 10: 561

Omodei MS, Delmanto LR, Carvalho-Pessoa E, et al. Association between pelvic floor muscle strength and sexual function in postmenopausal women. *Journal of Sexual Medicine* 2019; 19(12): 1938–1946

Panay N, Palacios S, Bruyniks N, et al. Symptom severity and quality of life in the management of vulvovaginal atrophy in postmenopausal women. *Maturitas* 2019 Jun 125: 55–61

Samuels JB, Garcia MA. Treatment to external labia and vaginal canal with CO_2 laser for symptoms of vulvovaginal atrophy in postmenopausal women. *Aesthetic Surgery Journal* 2019 Jan 1; 39(1): 83–93

Scavello I, Maseroli E, Di Stasi V, et al. Sexual health in menopause. *Medicina* 2019; Sep 2 33(9) pii: E559

Simon JA, Kagan R, Archer DF, et al. TX-004HT clinically improves symptoms of vulvar and vaginal atrophy in postmenopausal women. *Climacteric* 2019; 22(4): 412–418

Sparavigna A, Caputo A, Natoli A, et al. A randomised single-blind placebo-controlled study of a Visnadine Emulgel formulation on healthy postmenopausal women. *Minerva Ginecologica* 2019; 71(5): 353–358

Thomas HN, Hamm M, Hess R, et al. "I want to feel like I used to feel": a qualitative study of causes of low libido in postmenopausal women. *Menopause* 2020 Mar; 27(3): 289–294

INDEX

ABOUT THE AUTHOR

Maryon Stewart is a world-renowned healthcare expert who is referred to as the pioneer of the natural menopause movement. With more than twenty-eight years of knowledge and expertise, she coaches women in understanding the information, tools, and techniques needed to overcome the symptoms of menopause, to the point where many become completely symptom-free.

She has written twenty-eight popular self-help books published in the UK, coauthored a series of medical papers, written regular columns for numerous daily newspapers and magazines, and had her own TV and radio shows. Maryon was awarded a British Empire Medal in 2018 for services to drug education following her successful seven-year campaign at the Angelus Foundation, which she established in memory of her daughter Hester.

She spent over twenty years helping women through her clinic on Harley Street in London, but these days she helps women all over the world in one-on-one virtual consultations. In the summer of 2017, in response to demand from her Facebook group members, she launched her virtual Six-Week Natural Menopause Solution, a live online initiative, based on her successful five-month program. Maryon has recently established the Women's Wellbeing Movement in the United States. As well as making self-help films on menopause, Maryon is a regular contributor to the Femail column in the *Daily Mail*. In December 2018 she was voted one of the fifty most inspirational women in the UK by Femail. She had four children and now lives with her American husband in Florida and splits her time between home, New York, and London.

maryonstewart.com

maryonstewart.com/healthywiseandwell

enquiries@maryonstewart.com

Wikipedia: en.wikipedia.org/wiki/Maryon_Stewart

LinkedIn: www.linkedin.com/in/maryon-stewart-bem-b806634/

Facebook group — Midlife Switch: www.facebook.com/groups/
naturalmenopausemidlifeswitch/?ref=bookmarks

Twitter: @maryonstewart

Instagram: maryonstewartmenopause

YouTube: www.youtube.com/results?search_query=maryon+stewart